Understanding and Treating Mental Illness:

The Strengths and Limits of Modern Psychiatry

Understanding and Treating Mental Illness:

The Strengths and Limits of Modern Psychiatry

John M. Cleghorn, MD
and Betty Lou Lee
with Thirty-four Consultants

Hogrefe & Huber Publishers
Toronto • Lewiston, NY • Bern • Göttingen • Stuttgart

Library of Congress Cataloging in Publication Data

Understanding and treating mental illness: the strengths and limits of modern psychiatry / by John M. Cleghorn M.D.; with Betty Lou Lee.
p. cm.
"Sponsored by the Scientific Council, Canadian Psychiatric Association."
Includes bibliographical references.
ISBN 0-920887-73-2 : $19.95 (U.S.)
1. Psychiatry — Popular works. I. Cleghorn J. M. II. Canadian Psychiatric Association. Scientific Council.
RC460.U53 1991 90-4429
616.89 — dc20 CIP

Canadian Cataloguing in Publication Data

Main entry under title:
Understanding and treating mental illness
Includes bibliographical references.
ISBN 0-920887-73-2

1. Mental illness — Popular works. 2. Psychiatry — Popular works.
I. Cleghorn, J.M., 1933
II. Canadian Psychiatric Association. Scientific Council

RC460.U63 1991 616.89 C90-093853-6

12 Bruce Park Avenue
Toronto, Ontario M4P 2S3

P.O. Box 51
Lewiston, N.Y. 14092

Printed in Canada
by Hignell Printing Limited, Winnipeg, Manitoba

ISBN 0-920887-20-1
Hogrefe & Huber Publishers, Toronto • Lewiston, NY • Bern • Stuttgart
ISBN 3-456-81802-5
Hans Huber Publishers, Bern • Stuttgart • Toronto • Lewiston, NY

This book is dedicated to the memory of Dr. Sebastian Klaus Littman (1931–1986), a knowledgeable and caring psychiatrist, member of the Scientific Council of the Canadian Psychiatric Association, and Chairman of the Department of Psychiatry at the University of Calgary until his untimely death.

Published under the auspices of The Scientific Council, Canadian Psychiatric Association

Acknowledgements

This project has benefited from direct and efficient assistance by many people, including Max Fink MD, Carol Nadelson MD, of the American Psychiatric Press, Alex Saunders of the Canadian Psychiatric Association, and Yves Lamontagne MD, president of the Association Des Medecins Psychiatres du Quebec.

The authors and the Scientific Council also wish to recognize the role of the publishers in this project. Their willingness and ability to help us shape and develop this book has made significant improvements to the scope, presentation, and enjoyment of the final product.

Table of Contents

Preface

This is a very practical book. It is written for people with friends or relatives who are experiencing mental illness, as well as for other members of the general public interested in just how far our knowledge has developed in the area of psychiatry. As a result, it may also be helpful for experts in allied health professions who would benefit from an update on our technical capabilities in the mental health area.

The motivation for this project stems from the fact that there have been very substantial changes throughout this field in recent years, and as a result many people are likely to still have a somewhat incomplete view of where things now stand. In particular, this area of medicine has been dramatically maturing beyond arguments among the various well known schools of thought which existed in the past, and into a more factually oriented clinical science that is concerned with developing and implementing treatments which can be objectively shown to produce practical benefits.

In order to obtain the very best available information, numerous experts in this field were invited to explain the current state of knowledge with respect to the disorders in which they specialize. The resulting manuscripts were then passed on to an award-winning science writer, Betty Lou Lee, who succeeded in translating sometimes obscure professional language into understandable and yet intriguing English. The result is a factual, up-to-date, and interesting account of where we stand in our ability to recognize and treat mental health problems.

Several themes are evident throughout this book. One is that we are indeed making progress in this field, partly due to the assistance of researchers in the neurosciences and chemistry, as well as various technicians who are developing ever more powerful equipment which we can use to both identify and solve diverse psychiatric problems. The second general point which becomes clear is that many mental and emotional problems are turning out to have direct physical causes, or at least physical components. These discoveries are very helpful because they imply a much greater future ability to treat or prevent many types of disorders which are now regarded as largely emotional or "mental." A third theme is that psychological, social and behavioral methods of providing treatment and care augment the effectiveness of medical methods, and are often very effective by themselves for the less severe problems. A fourth important point in this book is that the costs to society which stem from mental illness are staggering, and therefore the benefits which we would reap from enabling perhaps millions of people to greatly improve their personal well-being and social productivity would likewise be enormous. As a result, almost strictly as an economic proposition, devoting greater resources to this area of social concern has a high potential to repay very substantial dividends, in terms of hard tax dollars saved, but also with respect to greater productivity, national competitiveness, and certainly quality of life for the former patients, as well as their families, friends, and colleagues.

While great progress has been made in the recent past, this book also reveals that we still need to develop additional techniques in order to better care for and prevent the very painful and costly disorders discussed in this book. In many cases changes in existing funding and regulatory policies in the US, Canada, and elsewhere would be very helpful. In addition, greater direct financial support is needed to also put existing knowledge into practice in order to help the mentally ill. Fortunately, many new techniques are now available to detect causes and create cures, but nonetheless more funds are required to support our investment in research, which is as crucial as it is highly productive.

J.M. Cleghorn, MD
Chairman (1983–1990) Scientific Council,
Canadian Psychiatric Association
Professor Emeritus and Past Chairman,
Department of Psychiatry McMaster University
University Coordinator (1975-83) of Mental Health
Services Hamilton-Wentworth Dist. Health Council
Professor of Psychiatry, University of Toronto

Chapter 1

An Introduction to the Challenges, the Treatments, and the Team

Psychiatric and psychological problems usually develop quite slowly. As a result, families with a person becoming mentally ill often cannot tell the difference between bad, sad or just plain weird, especially at the very beginning of the problem. In time they often come to blame themselves for the distress of their loved ones: "I guess I have always been too hard on him," is one common phrase, and "Maybe we never paid enough attention to her," is another.

Unfortunately, mental illnesses come in such a wide variety of alternatives that they do not lend themselves to a simple definition. It can also be quite difficult to diagnose these problems accurately. As with other complicated medical situations, it is crucial to thoughtfully consider the possible causes, the diverse symptoms, onset, course of the disease, and the response to various treatments.

Some mental problems, such as Alzheimer's Disease, clearly involve physical disorders of the brain. Damaged brain cells can be seen through a microscope and are often recognized as specifically different from normal cells. Indeed, many of these diseases which we now regard as emotional problems may well turn out to have direct physical causes, generally involving biochemical imbalances. For example, there is some tentative evidence that Alzheimer's Disease may be caused by an excessive buildup of aluminum in the brain. Various addictions, such as those to alcohol, caffeine, heroin or nicotine may be triggered by an oversupply of some enzyme or peptide which is not yet fully understood. Other problems, such as manic-depression, with its wild alterations in mood, or schizophrenia with its thought disturbances often causing massive incoherence, have long been thought to be genetically inherited. In the future, many illnesses will be more easily understood by the presence of an identified abnormal gene.

On the other hand, some psychiatric disorders are an extreme of a characteristic that occurs to a lesser degree in all people, and which in a severe form can be labelled an illness. Some would say that this is the case for anxiety, phobias, and panic attacks. A scale of "Five Ds" conveniently distinguishes types of problems:

- Dissatisfaction
- Demoralization
- Distress
- Disability
- Disease

So far, no unique gene detection or lab test can distinguish among these levels of severity. The less that is known about a disease, the more vague and bizarre the theories about it tend to be. This is somewhat akin to the fanciful explanations and treatments that were common for fever before the discovery of bacteria. However, when dissatisfaction, demoralization and distress are not accompanied by disease and disability then a change in circumstances or learning new ways to solve problems may be what is required (see pages 8-9 and 18-20). However, if there is disability and evidence of disease, then one of the psychiatric disorders described in this book may be present.

*** Prevalence

Psychiatric disorders involving distress and disability and often disease are extraordinarily common — much more so than most people suspect. They are a major public health problem, partly because of their high incidence, but also because of the incredible amount of both private and public resources which are employed to deal with them, even though there is considerable agreement that not yet enough is being done.

Many studies have shown that about one out of every five people in North America will experience what could be called a psychiatric disorder sometime during his or her lifetime. This figure has been a consistent finding in a number of large investigations over the years. The most recent research on adults, sponsored by the U.S. National Institute of Mental Health, was published in 1984 and involved 3,000 people in three cities. Drug abuse disorders were the most common, affecting 15 to 18 per cent of the population. A remarkable two-thirds of these people abused alcohol, and one-third were involved with other drugs. But even without considering substance abuse, 20 per cent had experienced another type of psychiatric disorder at some time.

Remarkably, one in eight persons will actually be hospitalized for some form of mental illness during their lifetime, and

Figure 1.1
Trends in Suicide Rates in the USA 1950-1985

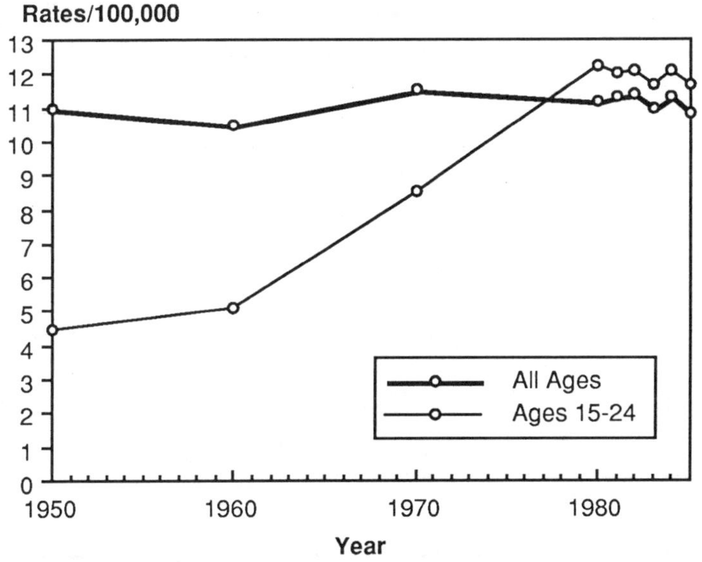

Source: National Center for Health Statistics, in: *Report of the Secretary's Task Force on Youth Suicide, Volume 1.* US Department of Health and Human Services, Public Health Service.

psychiatric problems are the second leading cause of general hospital admissions among those 20 to 44 years old. In addition, suicide is the second leading cause of death of persons aged 15 to 39. Even worse, for those in the age group 15-24 the rate has increased dramatically compared to the situation in 1950. Figures 1.1 to 1.4 show the variation in suicide rates by gender, country, age, and for the Canadian cases also by age in which death occurred.

Hospital costs alone for people in North America with mental illness are more than a $18 billion each year, and far more people are treated outside hospitals than in them.

The additional costs of unemployment and a wide variety of social services for the mentally ill and their families are undoubtedly much higher. Therefore the potential benefits to society from solving, "curing" or better yet preventing these problems would be enormous, and merely the hard dollar tax savings to citizens would be in the billions of dollars.

One of the most troubling aspects of mental health problems

Figure 1.2
US & Canadian Suicide Rates: 1955 – 1987
Gender Differences

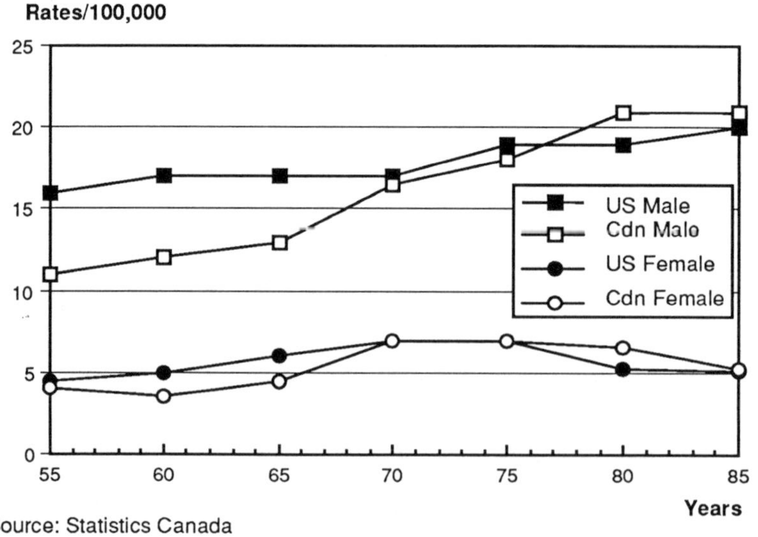

Source: Statistics Canada

Figure 1.3
Suicide Rates in Canada 1950 – 1988
Males by Age and Year of Death

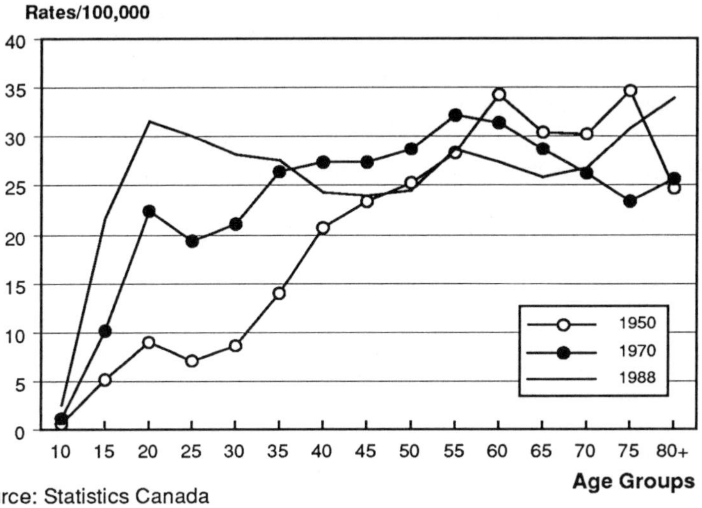

Source: Statistics Canada

Figure 1.4
Suicide in Canada 1950 – 1988
Females by Age and Year of Death

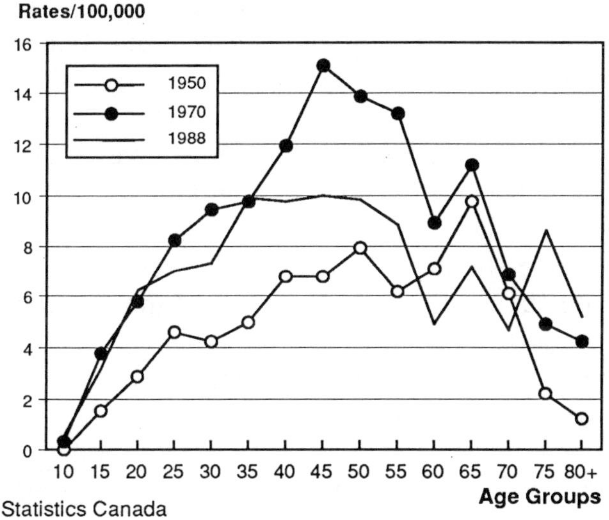

Source: Statistics Canada

Table 1.1
Mental Health Facilities in the USA: 1987

Number of Facilities	Inpatient Beds (1,000)	Inpatient Rate Per 100,000 Population	Expenditures $US Billions	Patient Care Staff (1,000)
4,747	268	99.4	18.5	346

Sources: U.S. National Institutes of Mental Health, Statistical Note Series, Statistical Abstract of the USA, 1990.

is that they often begin at an early age — late adolescence and early adulthood — which means that they interfere with education and employment, completely derailing an otherwise happy and productive future. The high degree of disability which is often involved over the many years, indeed decades, that these illnesses often persist, also compound the vast social costs incurred.

Yet far outweighing all these financial costs, and completely beyond the calculation of economics, is the cost in human misery and suffering:

- the young schizophrenic who must give up plans for a highly productive career in engineering

- the little children of a manic-depressive who can not understand why Daddy is "acting funny" again

- the wife who watches in despair as Alzheimer's Disease robs her of her husband

- the agoraphobic bereft of all social contacts outside the house

In addition, while we like to think of childhood as being happy and carefree, the young are far from immune to mental disorders. A major and comprehensive study of this subject was done in Ontario, Canada, in 1983. This project involved collecting some 2.5 million pieces of data on 3,300 children aged 4 to 16. The results showed that a remarkable 18 percent of them had one of the four most common emotional disturbances of childhood. These include:

- conduct disorder, with its chronic breaking of rules, lying, cheating and fighting

- hyperactivity, with its short attention span and impulsiveness

- emotional disorder with symptoms of anxiety and depression

- somatization (from the Greek word for body), where the child is seen by others and herself as sickly and delicate, or has many physical complaints such as pains or dizzy spells for which no physical cause can be found

The first two problems are most common in boys, the last two in girls.

The 18 percent figure in this study is similar to the results found in similar investigations carried out in the United States, Puerto Rico, and New Zealand.

An important related observation from the study showed that although the Province of Ontario spent $400 million on services related to childhood mental disorders in 1983, five out of six children with these problems had not received any mental health or social services at all in the previous six months.

A major study reported in early 1990 by the Bank Street College of Education in New York, showed that barely one-third of the school children in the USA who are emotionally disturbed are getting into programs which could help them. It was found that

42% of such disturbed children drop out of school, and overall between 3% and 5% of the elementary school population can be identified as emotionally disabled. In addition, the study also showed that most of the programs which these children do get into are aimed largely at maintaining classroom stability and silence, rather than solving the underlying problems involved.

* * * Emotional Problems of Everyday Life

Although the reported figures for mental illness are very high, a much larger number of people think they are sometimes affected with emotional problems which cause three of the D's listed on page 2 — Demoralization, Dissatisfaction and Distress. For example, many people experience "anxiety" to the point they feel they are coming apart and cannot stand the pressure they are

Figure 1.5
Number of Mental Health Professionals by Major Categories

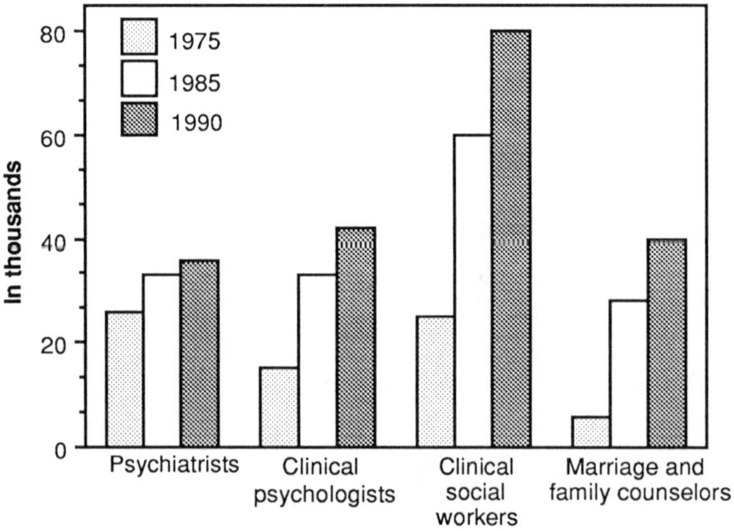

Source: American Psychiatric Association

under, but for most people these crises are not disabling, and they are only temporary.

Almost everyone has days of feeling down, anxious, unenthusiastic, and definitely unfriendly. Most people, however, who are considered "well adjusted" can handle these problems in rational and logical ways, such as by talking to friends or confidants, or doing something that usually makes them feel better, which often involves doing something that they do well, as this serves to restabilize confidence. When seriously troubled, of course many people find it very helpful to discuss their problems with a religious adviser.

Because we are social and biological creatures, these feelings of occasional emotional distress are quite natural, and require that we turn to those we know for help. We cannot entirely avoid these periodic low key crises any more than we can completely escape from cold viruses.

When you have a physical illness, and your grandmother's remedy, your friends' advice, your family doctor's efforts and time itself do not help, you start thinking of a specialist. With a mental illness, especially regarding more severe cases, the most highly qualified specialist, in terms of medical and scientific training is a psychiatrist, but of course there are several other groups of professionals who also deal with problems of mental and emotional health. Data for the USA show considerable growth in the number of professionals in this general field, even since only 1975.

The training and licensing requirements involved with these various professional categories vary quite widely, both between Canada and the USA, and within the states and provinces as well. Since this book is about the more severe disorders which may involve disease, distress and disability, we will focus on psychiatrists, whose aim is to understand and treat such disorders.

*** *Just What is a Psychiatrist?*

Someone with this title is a medical doctor who is a specialist in assessing and treating mental illness. He or she has the training and skills to diagnose and treat people with serious disturbances of mood, memory, thinking, perception, belief and behavior. Psychiatrists are able to give an expert opinion in a courtroom environment when called on to do so, and they are also legally able to prescribe a wide variety of medications.

After a would-be psychiatrist finishes medical school and obtains an M.D. degree, the next step is a one-year internship in medicine, surgery and other medical fields. This is followed by four years as a resident or apprentice in a hospital setting under the supervision of experienced psychiatrists. At this point the candidate must pass examinations on a broad range of medical and psychiatric subjects, and demonstrate a clear ability to assess, treat and improve the well being of patients. During this process the physician is closely observed by two senior colleagues who come from different university hospital settings than the ones in which the resident has trained.

People are often confused about the difference between a psychiatrist, a psychologist and the other mental health specialists. Psychologists earn a Master of Science or Ph.D. degree, which is followed by an internship of one or two years. They may have the title "doctor" by virtue of their Ph.D., but they are not physicians. They cannot, for example, prescribe medications. However, they do have intensive training in research methods, often more thorough than medical doctors. They are trained in such fields as personality assessment, counseling, or behavioral and cognitive therapies, and the scientific rationale for these approaches.

However, the word "therapist" is quite a general term for anyone offering therapy. There are many kinds of professionals from a wide variety of schools and training experiences who are called therapists, but in most areas, there is legally nothing to prevent people from simply declaring themselves therapists, regardless of the strengths or weaknesses of their qualifications. The laws in most places simply restrict the prescription of medications to medical doctors. Thus the person seeking therapy is in the difficult position of having to make a judgement about the adequacy of a therapist without the knowledge that a licensing body has approved of him or her. The characteristics of good therapists are described on page 20.

Fortunately, professional psychiatrists, psychologists and other counselors can be found in most areas of North America, and altogether they have at hand a considerable repertoire of techniques which can be applied to help treat many mental problems.

*** A Very Brief History

In the past, societies have had great difficulty understanding mental illness. In the early 1600s, the individuals with these problems were believed to be possessed by evil spirits, and they were simply burned at the stake as witches. By the early 19th century, different countries had evolved a variety of alternative approaches. In France and Germany, mental illnesses were regarded as physical disorders of the brain, and those who suffered from them were admitted to hospitals, where psychiatrists and neurologists worked together to try to understand the disease processes involved. By contrast, in England such problems were considered related to cycles of the moon, so the victims were called lunatics, from the Latin "luna" for moon. The Quakers tried to help them in a civilized and humane way, and established lunatic asylums. In particular, the Lunacy Act of 1890 provided humane confinement, but not treatment.

In 19th-century North America the mentally ill were regarded as sick and asylums were built for them, usually away from urban centers on farm land that was tilled by the patients themselves. The psychiatrists in charge of them were called "alienists." At their best these institutions were humane and peaceful; at their worst, they were "snake-pits" and "loony bins." The history of mental hospitals has been a cyclical one, with periods of humane care and high ideals, followed by eras of corruption and underfunding, sprinkled with periods of reform movements.

Generally the population of public mental hospitals continued to grow until about 30 years ago, at which point in the USA there were more than 550,000 patients in state and county facilities. Since that peak, various legal decisions and changes in treatments, especially the development of psychotropic medications, have reduced this figure to about 100,000.

Although it seems difficult for us to believe in the 1990s, it was not until the middle of this century that enhancements in the communications media allowed the public in general to develop greater awareness of how psychological factors can influence behavior. We now regard it as natural to speak of "Freudian slips," and to periodically undertake armchair psychoanalysis of why friends and relations act the way they do. Partly because of the growing sophistication and increasingly informed nature of the public, there grew a greater comprehension of the emotional dimension of everyday life, the needs of children, the normal crises and tribulations of human development, and the distorted

Figure 1.6
Number of Patients in State and County Hospitals in the USA

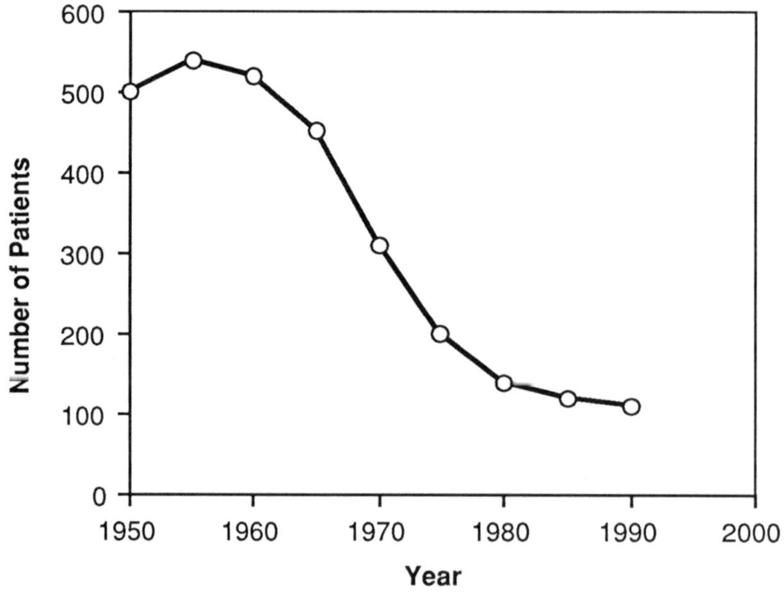

Source: US National Institute of Mental Health

way in which we sometimes come to regard each other and have trouble communicating.

These understandings apply to normal people, to normal people with troubles, and to some people with troubled backgrounds and misfortunes in early development. Psychological insights are useful in learning how to live in a less anxious and more satisfying way. But they aren't much help by themselves in treating the severe psychiatric disorders described in this book, any more than an understanding of what pneumonia is and what causes it is of help when someone is having difficulty breathing. After a point, it becomes time to call in a specialist.

Fortunately, as a result of many scientific advances over the past 30 years, the modern psychiatrist's work involves much more than the stereotypical couch, or endless debates among proponents of various schools of psychiatric thought. Fortunately, the science of psychiatry has evolved steadily to where now the major areas of importance include not only psychology but neuroscience, electronic imaging, modern psychopharmacology and many avenues of research to evaluate the effectiveness of treatment. These days the majority of patients are in fact treated in clinics or doctors' offices. General hospitals have psychiatric wards where the average stay is about one month. In addition, admission to a specialized psychiatric hospital is no longer a life sentence — the average stay is now less than two months, compared to 10, 20 or even 40 years which characterized psychiatric hospitalizations in the past, especially those involving schizophrenia.

Specific disorders of the mind and brain are the special interest of psychiatrists, but the brain certainly does not sit in isolation from the body in any situation. For better or worse, there is a constant interaction — just think how differently you think, feel and act when you have a bad case of the flu.

One aspect of the psychiatrist's knowledge is physical — the biology of the brain and what can go wrong with it; how defects in genes can cause cells to function in certain ways; the influences of chemical messengers in the brain; and how to use the latest technology and methods to deal with these problems, among others.

But over the last hundred years psychiatrists and psychologists also have developed skills and specific techniques to assess a person's ability to cope with life, and to learn new methods of solving problems, or to pinpoint what has gone wrong in learning how to live comfortably and productively.

Despite the historical importance and contribution of modern technology, the psychiatrist first takes into consideration the social context in which a patient lives, and the many effects this can have. One's social context is of course made up of many circles of influences in one's social network. One person may be depressed because she is solely responsible for several children and has no one to lean on or talk to. Another may become depressed because he carries a gene that will not allow the brain to produce enough chemicals to maintain a good mood. If treatment is to be effective, it is essential to distinguish between these two situations.

The development of this field has also shown that it is important to consider the cultural context of a patient's situation, since abnormal behavior is defined in different ways in different settings. People from one culture who are upset are more likely to complain of physical symptoms; those of another, emotional ones. Regardless of the definitions, numerous studies during this century, involving many different cultures around the world, have shown that 15 to 20 percent of most every population is prone to mental health disorders involving clearly abnormal behavior.

Over roughly the last 100 years psychiatrists have become more expert at assessing personality, i.e., those patterns of thought and behavior that are unique to each of us, and which are the outcome of inherited factors, family influences, and the impact of significant events. Many studies during this century have also helped psychiatrists better understand how people respond to physical or psychological disabilities.

For example, someone who was a timid child of elderly, bookish parents, did well in school and avoided all sports, might respond to depression with symptoms of withdrawal, guilt and self-depreciation. His neighbor, a noisy, outgoing, athletic man from a large and gregarious family, might respond with irritability, violence, and alcoholism.

*** Assessment and Treatment Alternatives

The purpose of this book is to explain what is known, and also what is not yet known, about psychiatric disorders, and what kinds of treatments have been clearly proven to work. Such information is important for people who are making choices about the kind of professional help they or their relatives may need, now or in the future.

But in addition, agencies that pay for health services increasingly demand information on the effectiveness of specific treatments, in order to help weigh the potential benefits against hard-dollar insurance and taxpayer costs. These agencies increasingly refuse to pay for treatments that are known to simply not work. But on the other hand, when there is no known treatment it is a doctor's job to keep searching for workable solutions and to not give up on a patient.

The first step is to take a thorough history of the patient, which begins with an in-depth interview to detect what kind of distress motivated the person to seek help at this time. What recent events have occurred in his or her life? Has there been a change in the way life is experienced? Is the distress impairing work performance or family life? What was the optimal level of functioning in the past, and how has this changed? Is there evidence of impaired brain function, such as severely reduced memory? Has there been exposure to toxic substances, or a recent severe infectious disease?

The second step is often a careful neurological assessment, perhaps involving an electroencephalogram (EEG), which reports the level of electrical activity in different parts of the brain, or an electronic scan showing the anatomy and structures of the brain itself. The most common scan is "computerized axial tomography" (CAT), but a more precise one, called "magnetic resonance imaging" (MRI) is gaining popularity. Remarkably, this technique gives a picture of the brain almost as accurate as that seen by examining tissue at an autopsy. These various technologies are discussed further in Chapter 2.

The third step, if there clearly does not seem to be a

medically related brain function problem, involves the pursuit of various psychological issues:

- What does the patient think is wrong
- What he or she thinks caused the problem
- What is the greatest concern about it.

A number of questions are frequently used to explore these issues, for example:

- Are there repetitive thoughts which precede episodes of anxiety or depression?
- Does the distress occur in particular circumstances?
- Does any relative or acquaintance have this problem?
- Has there been a hazardous life event, such as a major accident or a loss of a loved one or personal property?
- Has there been a major developmental stage that has caused a life crisis: graduation, leaving home, marriage, divorce or retirement?
- With female patients in particular, has there been a history of abuse?
- Does the person have low self-esteem? Does he or she feel well put together, with a solid sense of identity, a meaningful past and a reliable future, or is there a sense of fragmentation and falling apart?
- Does the family want anything to change, and what are its needs for stability? Is there a circle of friends, and people who can be relied on for support? Is the patient a member of a self-help group?
- Do eating habits vary considerably from the person's social group? What about alcohol and street drug use?

These are just a sampling of some of the questions that must be answered to make a reasonably accurate assessment. In addition, family members may also be interviewed, and psychological tests as well as medical laboratory examinations may be required before a clear-cut diagnosis can be made. The various major psychiatric problems which might be discovered are reflected in the chapter headings of this book.

With the patient's help, the doctor will try to find out what predisposed the person to this illness, what precipitated it, and what actually keeps it going. Are there important factors mitigating against improvements? Are there particular strengths or protective factors which keep the person functioning at a better level than might otherwise be expected, such as a good marital relationship, particular talents or abilities?

The fourth step, after all these data have been carefully assembled, and the diagnosis made, is to implement a treatment appropriate to the illness involved. Fortunately, there are many different kinds of psychiatric treatments, and quite a variety of combinations may be used for the same patient.

* * * *Types of Medications Used in the Treatment of Mental Illness*

Each of the following chapters deals in some detail with a specific mental illness, and reviews the various drugs which are most effective in each case. But it is worthwhile to present here an overview of the broad classes of treatments which are now available.

The Neuroleptic Medications. These are drugs which were introduced in North America only in 1954, by the eminent psychiatrist Heinz Lehmann. They have enabled many thousands of troubled people to live outside of hospitals, so that we no longer have many of the stereotypical asylums from centuries past. Because of their power, potential side effects, and often highly specific nature, these medications are used mainly in connection with psychotic disorders.

But these drugs only control symptoms — so far they do not cure. There is an urgent need, and the opportunity has never been better, for scientific research to go beyond the current generation of medications and develop more specific drugs with fewer side effects.

Anti-Depressants and Lithium. These are another group of effective medications which are not quick pep-me-ups, but drugs that slowly over several weeks alter depressed moods and the chemical imbalances within the brain which may generate them. They can actually cure, but they work so slowly that suffering is persistent and continues to create social and emotional cost. A greater understanding of brain chemistry and how mood can be altered more quickly would be a major contribution in this field.

Tranquillizers and Anxiolytics (Anti-Anxiety Agents). These widely used drugs have been very useful in helping people to control excessive anxiety. While they are very effective for treating severe problems of this kind as well as phobic disorders, they also carry a risk of addiction, and this is another area that cries out for research progress to develop effective medications.

*** Other Therapies

Psychotherapy. This form of treatment involves learning to solve one's emotional problems, which can cause severe dissatisfaction, demoralization and distress, by talking them out with a trained medical or non-medical therapist. Usually people learn to cope from their parents and friends, but some of us get stuck in ruts and repeat the same unhappy pattern over and over again, like the much-married woman whose every husband is an alcoholic.

Many problems of living are often reactions to milestones in the life cycle, such as birth, school entrance, marriages, divorce, retirement and death. What kind of reaction is normal depends on the culture, and the group or family in which a person lives. One family, for example, might think it normal for a daughter to become independent and pursue a career; another might expect her to remain at home and look after her younger siblings.

It is sometimes a long and arduous task to unlearn ineffective ways of solving problems and learn healthier ones, and it requires considerable skill by the therapist. But sometimes psychotherapy can be very brief and a tiny change can start a long term chain reaction.

For example, a young woman afraid to leave home for fear her sick mother cannot manage alone is torn between a desperate need for a life of her own, and her guilt about what may happen to her mother. She starts getting stomach pains and anxiety attacks, and can't leave the house. Her therapist acknowledges that it is normal for her to feel frustrated and angry in this situation, and this feedback helps to reduce some of her anxiety and guilt. In the second session, which includes her brothers and sisters, they suddenly realize that she is carrying all the burden, and decide to share their mother's care so the daughter can get a place of her own. Her anxiety then disappears.

There are many forms of psychotherapy, and many ways of taking part in it. Some are best done on a one-to-one basis, some involve the whole family, and others include groups of people sharing similar problems. Couples and families can get stuck in self-wounding cycles just like individuals can.

What is termed "dynamic" therapy involves regular sessions over varying lengths of time, in which the therapist tries to uncover the real person behind what might be a protective facade used as armor to ward off further hurt, or in other cases a loss of conscious awareness of events in the past which are too painful to remember. This form of therapy tries to develop insight into the internal emotional forces that are producing ineffective methods of coping. Its aim is to restore morale, increase self-assurance, and provide the understanding needed to choose effective ways of solving problems, as well as the ability to accept what truly cannot be changed.

Psychotherapy for these sorts of problems is particularly helpful. A brief treatment regime with this technique might involve weekly one-hour sessions for up to a year. Longer-term therapy is available in many centers, and might sometimes continue for several years.

Many people feel that they have been helped by psychoanalysis, but so far it has been impossible to scientifically evaluate its efficacy in the same way that other treatments have been assessed. Its effects are more subtle and difficult to measure, although they may be profound to the patient who has benefited. Unfortunately, this sort of psychiatric help, by itself, is not much use in treating the severe psychiatric disorders described in this book. People with extreme problems may also have other difficulties which psychoanalysis can help. Nevertheless, to use it alone for the treatment of a serious mental illness may be tantamount to helping a patient with a peptic ulcer based on insight regarding what causes it, while neglecting to call in a specialist who can treat it vigorously and effectively.

While there are people who can't get along with one another through no fault of either person, the same is true of therapists and patients. Sometimes it's just a case of character incompatibility. Just because one "match" does not work out doesn't mean another might not be successful. One should not write off psychotherapy after a single unproductive experience, any more than attempts to find a spouse should be stopped because a first date was disappointing.

There is more involved with psychotherapy than an expert doctor who knows that bacterium A calls for antibiotic X. It is a mixture of art and science. Therefore, it is only natural that there are a number of attributes in therapists which have been found over the decades to bring relatively good results.

Physicians who are especially good in this field are warm, caring, responsive and accepting. They should be reliable and keep promises, since many people in therapy have lost their ability to trust anyone at all because they have been hurt and disappointed so much in the past.

Since none of us is perfect, therapists should be aware of their own character and vulnerabilities. They should have respect for patients, and not treat them like children or idiots. In addition, they should have a realistic optimism about the improvements that can be expected. They should also have the strength to be flexible, to know when to talk and when to listen, to allow the patient to grow, and when the time comes, to let them go completely. Of course, the therapist should not be sexually or verbally abusive, judgmental, condescending or uncommunicative.

All these qualities are important because psychotherapy works not only by means of understanding or insight, but also through the quality of the relationship with the patient during the course of therapy. Being treated in certain ways can lead to healing, growth and development. While patients may experience hurts and disappointments with their therapists, as with other people in the past, understanding and overcoming these hurts allows the patient to become less vulnerable, and to develop better relationships in the future.

Cognitive Behavioral Therapy. This approach to solving emotional problems is based on the observation that thoughts can often determine feelings and actions. Rather than looking for emotional insight or a deeper understanding of the patient's childhood traumas, the therapy is specifically designed to directly change behavior patterns in a planned way. The therapist may work out a highly individualized behavioral "prescription" so that the patient learns ways of reversing spiraling waves of negative thinking, or the first signs of a panic attack.

Not surprisingly, some kinds of people respond better to one type of psychotherapy than another. The practical down-to-earth person who believes in action may be helped by learning new skills and techniques for managing self-defeating behavior, or ways of thinking. Those who are introspective or who have a deep sense of tradition and family history may prefer an approach which looks at family patterns over generations.

In addition, many modern women will be wary of an old-fashioned male-oriented psychotherapy. The women's movement has challenged the traditional roles of men and women, and norms for the roles of men and women are changing. Many therapists now no longer try to define normality by the old conventional roles.

Rehabilitation Therapy. This approach is used when basic living skills have not been developed or have been lost in the course of a major illness. Rehabilitation usually involves a new kind of learning, such as those skills needed to work more effectively, find a job, maintain a place to live, shop, or function well in an interview. Fortunately there are many programs for people with serious emotional illnesses which can help restore them to an independent life.

Electroconvulsive Therapy (ECT). This is the most controversial treatment in psychiatry, and its most frequent application is to cure severe depression. Much of the concern about this technique has been based on its excessive and inappropriate use in the past. ECT was often given without anesthetic, and attendants would hold a patient's arms and legs to prevent injury when a seizure occurred — a thoroughly frightening procedure. Now, patients are given a brief general anesthesia as well as medication to relax the muscles so that the limbs will not thrash about during the procedure. In spite of this, a recent survey in Great Britain showed that 50 to 60% of patients are afraid of this technique, even when it is carefully explained to them. Yet most agree to it, and sign a consent document that demonstrates they understand the treatment and its risks.

Many patients and their families are afraid of brain damage and the loss of memory. In the past there was slight memory loss, but this can be greatly reduced, if not eliminated, by placing the electrodes over the right side of the head, rather than the left where verbal memory is stored, in people who are right-handed.

Others are afraid of pain, which is generally minimal due to the anesthetic. In contrast, many psychiatrists tell their colleagues that they would want ECT treatments if they were ever caught in a depression, since they have witnessed the pain associated with this particular malady, and would want it over as quickly as possible.

These days ECT is mainly used for depressions that do not respond to anti-depressant medications. When used correctly, ECT is effective, safe, and it quite often does bring fast results, although it is not fully understood exactly why it works. Nonetheless it can be life-saving in situations where the person might commit suicide before drug medications could work. This approach is discussed further in chapter 3 regarding depression.

Surgery. The developer of an operation called a "frontal lobotomy" won a Nobel Prize because this procedure did effectively relieve suffering in the days before drugs and ECT. While some patients did relatively well, and were even able to continue professional work, many were left with a clear lack of emotional vitality. On the other hand, scarring of brain tissue resulted in epilepsy in some patients, and about 5% died as a result of brain hemorrhage caused by the surgery. Some became excitable and unable to control their emotions, still others required total care because of severe brain damage.

These varied and unpredictable outcomes were due to a lack of precision in the surgery, when some parts of the brain necessary for good functioning were damaged. When the technique was refined and tightly focused on particular parts of the frontal lobes, better results were achieved, but this entire approach was generally abandoned in the 1950s.

More broadly, neurosurgery in general is now widely used to deal with a variety of brain disorders, including those caused by tumors. Surgery is also employed to remove parts of the brain which cause seizures.

We may one day find that some of the brain cells which act as chemical factories can be replaced when they have become exhausted, or can be dampened down when they are over-producing. Little bits of brain tissue that secrete just the right amount and kind of chemical might be implanted. Current research in genetics and on brain tissue implantation in animals is promising, but human application will require tremendous scientific effort over the next few decades.

One interesting step in this direction is the recent development of a brain tissue bank, which is now being widely utilized by researchers.

Due to this facility, experts can study and compare the medical characteristics of healthy versus diseased brain tissue more readily than in the past. Many patients and their families are deciding to indeed participate in this program by allowing post mortem donations into this bank. Further details are available via McLean Hospital, 115 Mill Street, Belmont, MA 02178.

*** The Treatment Team

Serious mental illnesses often require a tightly coordinated group of mental health professionals working together to help the patient and his or her family with the difficult problems that disturbed behavior brings for all of them. Such treatment teams in adult and child psychiatry are composed of some or all of the following professionals.

Psychiatric Nurses usually have been women, but increasing numbers of men are going into this field, which involves taking either an R.N. at a community college and/or a bachelor's degree in nursing at a University. The latter is increasingly favored these days by the nursing profession itself. Following the completion of training, a person interested in psychiatric nursing might take special courses or begin an apprenticeship as an employed nurse on a psychiatric service, either inpatient or outpatient. Such nurses acquire great experience over several years of practice, and they become quite expert at assessing patients' problems and how to manage them. They also become knowledgeable about the use of drugs and their side effects, and actually carry out the care of patients on a day-to-day basis, usually with a doctor's supervision and also with doctors assuming the medical-legal risks and authority. An experienced psychiatric nurse is a highly skilled professional who can go on to leadership positions in clinics, and some enter private practice as well.

Social Workers are invaluable members of the assessment and treatment team. They have special expertise at understanding persons in their social context. While many of them work in public sector agencies and on social policy teams in government, there are also clinical social workers who develop skills in case work and psychotherapy, and become expert at helping clients and families solve emotional problems. The basic training for these experts involves a minimum of a B.A. but also usually a Master's degree or a "Master of Social Work," usually known as an MSW, through which they develop a good understanding of community organization and the many, sometimes very complicated, sources of support for patients, particularly the poor and socially disadvantaged. They are expert at helping people with disabilities be placed in suitable residences, and in training programs to upgrade their skills. Social workers often begin their careers in the public sector, and sometimes later become private practitioners specializing in clinical work with marriage therapy, drug abuse, industrial psychology, and so on. Some also become clinic directors, in part because of their knowledge of how social systems work equips them to become administrators.

Occupational Therapists have special skills in assessing the specific assets and deficits of people with psychological, physical or developmental disabilities, and in helping them overcome these problems, as well as learn alternative ways of coping with mental and physical challenges. In addition, they can help patients learn how to utilize leisure time in a constructive way, and thus develop specific methods of coping with their distress. They are also able to assess the occupational potential of a patient, and to set up graduated steps of increasing responsibility. This may be done in either hospital or in community settings. Experts in this field usually acquire a bachelor's or a master's degree in occupational therapy from a university. Much of the academic training involves the science of anatomy and related fields, with an increasing emphasis on the many new electronically assisted techniques which are increasingly available to help patients in this area.

Child Care Workers usually acquire a diploma from a community college or a bachelor's degree from a university, during which they learn a great deal about how children develop, with emphasis on the psychological and cognitive stages involved, and how families function. As a result they are often quite well equipped to understand both healthy and disturbed children, and to participate extensively in their care via residential treatment settings, hospitals, or community daycare centers. Some child care workers go on to take degrees in different fields and to become administrators, nurses, or therapists.

Psychologists, described on page 10, also have a crucial role in assessment and treatment.

*** Treatment and Release Paradox

As the number of people held in mental hospitals has declined dramatically over the last 40 years, a growing number of people who were former patients have had trouble adjusting to community life. In many cases where strong family or friend support systems have been absent, the result has been unemployment, homelessness, and hunger. Understandably some of these people can sometimes appear a bit unnerving to normal people who encounter them walking down the street.

Partly because of the sensationalism which the media have applied to isolated crimes committed by former mental patients, the public often reacts to these people with fear, and the result is an effective social isolation. As a result, in an era of greatly increased knowledge about mental illness, the prejudice against its victims appears to be remaining quite strong. For example, in a recent study in the US, mental illness was ranked as the worst of 21 possible disabilities which one could have, and ex-convicts were rated higher on a scale of social acceptance than former mental patients. A California study found that only 17% of the respondents agreed with the statement that “mental patients are not dangerous.”

Occasionally social stereotypes do have some vague validity. Anyone who thinks that a tourist from Japan will behave the same as one from Texas has clearly never been a host to either. But in the case of the mentally ill, the dangerousness factor is just not supported by the facts. Most such people are in fact withdrawn, timid, and themselves quite anxious about others. Repeated studies have shown that fewer than 2% of mental patients pose any threat to society. Some nonetheless feel that the potential unpredictability of these people is a reason to fear them, though they are usually dependably passive.

In contrast, drunk drivers are some of the most predictably dangerous people in North America, and account for about 30,000 deaths each year. Yet tolerance, and even sympathy for these individuals has remained remarkable over the decades, though this appears to be changing now.

Perhaps as the research of psychiatrists proceeds, and the public becomes more well informed, concern about the dangerousness of the mentally ill, and the social isolation which accompanies it, will diminish. Those with polio, diabetes, or Parkinson’s disease are not feared or isolated, and indeed are generally given sympathy and support. As it becomes increasingly clear that many mental illnesses are due to underlying physical problems which simply generate odd behavior patterns, the level of understanding for these victims may also increase.

A step in this direction is reflected in a recent survey undertaken by the National Restaurant Association, the first trade group to ever study employment experience with the mentally restored. The results showed that over 75% of the employers involved rated these people "as good or better" than their co-workers in terms of motivation, quality of work, and job tenure.

*** For Further Information

Some of the chapters in this book have references for getting help or more detailed information on the disorder being discussed. Initial information about the services available in your community can often be obtained from your family doctor, the local public health agency, or the Mental Health Association, listed in the white pages of the phone book. In addition, the local library can also be remarkably helpful.

A little information can go a long way when you have a troubled relative and do not understand what's wrong. But one note of caution. There is a condition called "medical students' disease," where people often seem to develop every medical problem they study. It is possible to find in yourself symptoms of almost any ailment. Everyone has had a headache, but few people have brain tumors. We all know someone who has felt depressed, paranoid or panicky at some time, but it is important to be careful and not draw too many immediate conclusions about your own situation, or the mental health of your friends, upon a first reading of the following chapters.

Chapter 2

Schizophrenia

This is one of the most puzzling, and expensive, diseases known to occur among humans, and it afflicts men and women equally. It occurs in about 1% of the population in North America, and in the USA alone there are some 2.5 million victims of this condition. Canada accounts for another 260,000 such patients. Schizophrenia accounts for a remarkable $25 billion to $30 billion in annual health care costs in the USA. On any given day about 25% of the total people in hospitals throughout the country are schizophrenics.

If a total cure for this disease were miraculously found tomorrow, the cost savings to taxpayers would be remarkable. This disease fills more beds in hospitals, nursing homes and long-term care facilities than any other single illness. Unfortunately it usually hits people just as they are getting started in life, in their late teens or early 20s.

The term comes from the Greek words for split and mind, and many mistakenly think the disease is one involving either a split personality — Jekyll and Hyde, or a case of multiple personalities, such as in The Three Faces of Eve, where several distinct identities develop, often unknown to each other, and often as an attempt to "escape" from severe childhood abuse.

But in contrast to these stereotypes, the split is instead with reality. Schizophrenics spend much of their time in another world, where voices inside their heads may comment on things they do and think, or tell them what to do, or carry on conversations among themselves. They may see, hear, touch, feel and taste things that aren't there. They lack the sense of control over themselves which most of us feel most of the time. They often imagine that they are being controlled by beings from another world, or that enemies are monitoring them through telephone or radio lines.

In many of these individuals, the thinking processes have become so disjointed that their talk no longer makes sense to anyone. They can suddenly express feelings of elation, anxiety, bewilderment, sadness or anger that have nothing to do with the circumstances they are in.

Victims of this disease have trouble sorting out where reality begins and fantasy ends. During acute episodes, when overcome by terror or anger, a small percentage may become violent and harm themselves or other people, but for the most part they are withdrawn and quiet, and rather sadly harmless. Because their actions, talk and appearance can be bizarre, frustrated friends and family often abandon them to their delusions and hallucinations, further adding to their withdrawal and isolation.

Margaret Gibson, an author and a schizophrenic, gives a glimpse of that other world and the terrors it can hold:

> *There are certain chairs one must not sit on, knocks on doors when there is no one there ... I have seen Satan, an angel disguised as a taxi driver, and run through the snow in stockinged feet with my three-year-old son because it was not 1976 any longer ... Only my son and I were left alive, searching for the underground where we would be safe with others who were not the enemy.*

The early stages of the disease may not be very dramatic. Family members may describe the person as "not himself:" he may be more introverted and withdrawn, and have difficulty coping with family, school or work. He may lack drive or interest, or have trouble concentrating. But these rather vague symptoms can be caused by anything from depression to smoking marijuana, so they should not, in themselves, be considered to be schizophrenia without a careful professional assessment.

About 25% of the people with schizophrenia find that their symptoms never become really severe. Roughly 50% more can be treated with medications, which include such names as Prolixin,

Haldol and Mellaril. However, these drugs can often cause side effects which can be quite severe. The remaining 25% are generally resistant to medication, or indeed most any form of therapy, and they often suffer long term relegation to isolation and hospitalization.

There are also more mild forms of schizophrenia in which the personality is not totally disorganized, and the individual appears fairly normal, but nonetheless the symptoms of the very severe form of the disease develop in the background. Here is an example:

> *In his late teens, Eric began to complain of a markedly diminished ability to concentrate, a sense of inner confusion, and an inability to control his thoughts. He began to spend most of his time in his bedroom, vacantly staring into space, and apparently not comprehending much of what was said to him, or suddenly fixing his attention on something like the lamp.*
>
> *By age 23, after two periods in a psychiatric hospital, he had been working for two years and was successfully maintained on a small dose of an antipsychotic drug, called perphenazine. But thinking he was better and no longer needed this medication, he stopped taking it. On his next routine clinic visit, his doctor noticed he seemed more anxious and less coherent, and persuaded him to start taking the medication again. But driving home, he became terrified when a traffic officer pointed at his car to wave him through an intersection. He then leapt out of the car, and raced back to the clinic saying the police were after him.*
>
> *He voluntarily agreed to go into a hospital for his own safety, and when he became less afraid, he explained that a customs officer had found his medication when he made a recent trip into the United States. He believed the officer had sent out an alert that he was trafficking in drugs, and that he would soon be jailed.*

On a higher dose of medication, he was able to leave the hospital after four weeks, but the ongoing drug therapy slowed him down, and he went back to work at a lower performance level than before. In another six months the medication could be reduced further and he became more energetic.

*** Causes

Over the centuries, there have been no shortage of explanations for this most disabling of mental illnesses. Possession by demons was a popular one. A century ago, masturbation was considered to be the cause, and later poor nutrition was the culprit. A few decades ago, parents were sent on guilt trips by being told that the disease was the result of the way they brought up the child. All these theories have been discarded.

At present, as in so many other areas of mental illness, several factors are thought to be involved, with significant variations among individuals. It is much more clear now that a predisposition to the disease may be inherited. If one parent has had a schizophrenic illness, the chance of the child developing this problem rises dramatically, from the normal one in a hundred, to one in 10. If both parents were schizophrenic, the risk jumps to about 45%. Interestingly, these higher risks hold even if the child is adopted by non-schizophrenic parents. Since this is a promising area for finding the explanation to this disease, it is important to discuss these risks a bit further.

Because the majority of schizophrenics' children do not develop the disease, and the majority of schizophrenics do not have schizophrenic parents, there have to be more factors involved than just genetic bad luck. Complications before or during birth, and/or head injuries have been clearly identified as risk factors. It is also well known that stress can make the symptoms worse, and schizophrenics may have especially poor coping mechanisms, but there is no formal scientific evidence that stress itself has a clear role in actually promoting development of the disease.

New techniques for looking at the structure and workings of the brain are revealing some differences in schizophrenics, and most psychiatrists believe that it results from complex physical disorders of brain function. A recent report from the National Institute of Mental Health has provided the best evidence to date that schizophrenia is a physiological brain disorder, and not just a psychological condition. Using 15 pairs of identical twins, of whom one was schizophrenic and the other normal, scientists discovered subtle anatomical differences in their brain cavities. Certain of the cavities or "ventricles" were enlarged in the mentally ill twins, while, in contrast, the brain regions involved with memory, emotion and decision making were reduced in size. These differences indicated that the tissue had shrunk, or developed abnormally. Since the twins studied were identical genetically, this study shows that clearly other factors than heredity are involved in schizophrenia — perhaps viral infections, oxygen deprivation, or traumas which affect the development of neural tissue.

In particular, it turns out that some areas of the brain which control movement and emotional response have an abnormally high number of receptors for dopamine, an important chemical messenger. In 1974 Dr. Philip Seeman of the University of Toronto discovered that this situation particularly applies to some schizophrenic patients.

Dopamine is one of a group of chemicals called "neurotransmitters," needed for nerve cells to communicate with one another. When an electrical impulse is travelling along the dendrite or tentacle of a nerve cell, a tiny amount of neurotransmitter is needed for it to bridge the gap, or synapse, between the dendrite of the neighboring nerve cell, as suggested in Figure 2.1.

Since this bit of physiology is quite important, several elements of this picture deserve an explanation. For example the axon is the nerve trunk line which carries electrical impulses rapidly from one place to another. Inside are microtubules involved in very slowly transporting substances which nourish the neuron. The term neuron includes both the axon and the cell body. Very critical chemical messengers, such as dopamine, are manufactured in the cell body, with energy generated in the mitochon-

Figure 2.1
Basic Physiology of Dendrite and Synapse Areas of Nerve Cells

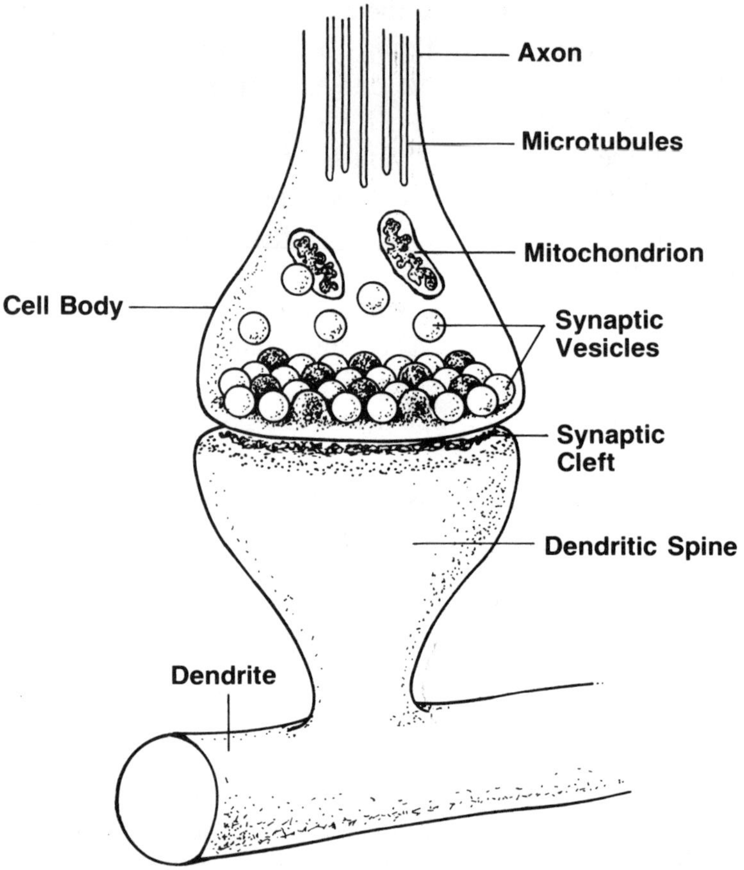

drion and stored in packets called vesicles. The synapse is the location of contact between nerve cells, a cleft into which the neurotransmitters are actually released.

Various drugs used for schizophrenia and other psychiatric disorders are designed to work directly with this anatomical reality. Some increase the body's release of a neurotransmitter, or in other cases act to reduce its action by blocking the receptor on the far side of the synapse. Other medications block the re-uptake of the neurotransmitter itself once it is released.

Antipsychotic drugs called "neuroleptics" have been carefully engineered to block the receptor on the neighboring nerve cell so that the electrical impulse cannot be transmitted. Figure 2.2 illustrates how the body manufactures dopamine, and the various intriguing elements which neuroleptics must therefore work against to achieve their aim.

Figure 2.2
Outline of Dopamine Generation and Neuroleptic Blocking Action

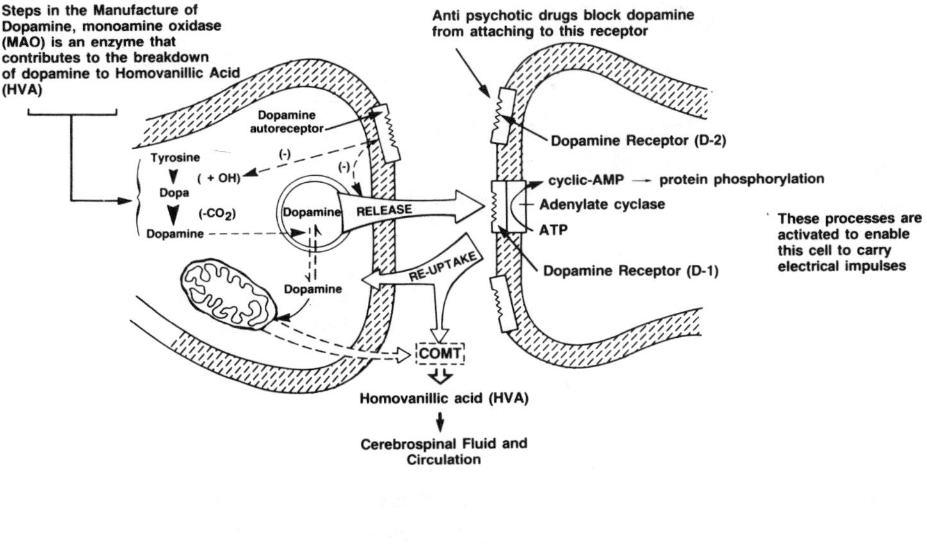

In the cell body, on the left, the steps in the manufacture of dopamine are shown. Tyrosine is a vitamin supplied in normal diets and it is transformed to dopamine, a chemical messenger involved in normal alertness and learning, which is produced in excess in schizophrenia. MAO (monoamine oxidase) is an enzyme that contributes to the breakdown of dopamine to HVA (homovanillic acid). Dopamine is normally released into the gap or synaptic cleft between the cell bodies and activates chemical processes which in turn lead to the transmission of electrical impulses in the neuron on the right side of the diagram.

In the case of schizophrenia, an overactive dopamine system may result in too much information reaching higher brain centers, so the messages get scrambled. Figure 2.3 shows dopamine neurons that originate deep in the middle of the brain and travel to higher centers in the frontal lobes.

Figure 2.3
Basic Overview of the Distribution of Dopamine Neurons

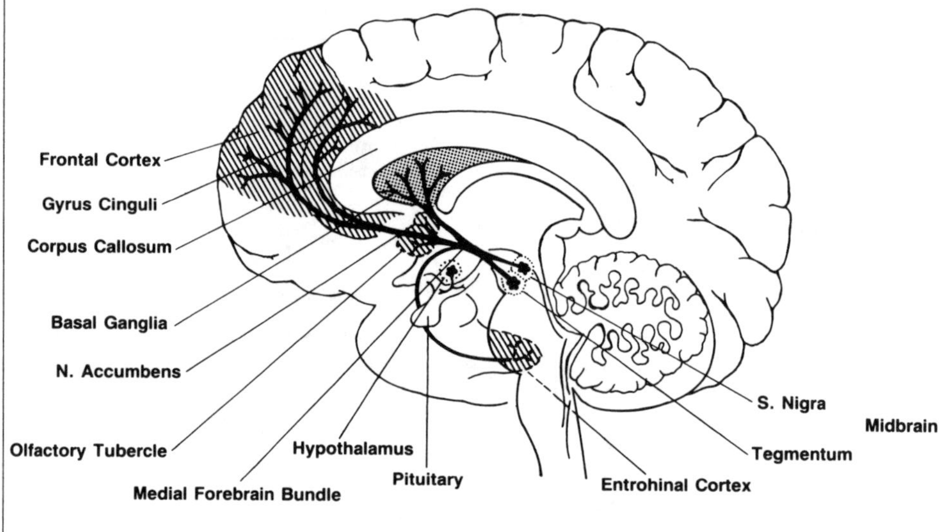

The distribution of dopamine neurons is illustrated by the dark lines in this diagram of the inside of the brain. The left is the front and the right is the back of the brain. This system of neurons may be faulty in schizophrenia, and the dopamine they secrete is blocked from activating other neurons by the antipsychotic drugs. The neurons travel to the frontal part of the cortex in which planning and attention are carried out in addition to other higher intellectual functions. They also travel to the gyrus cinguli, which is involved in attachment and communication between people, and to the basal ganglia which help in the coordination of movement and thinking.

*** Treatment

From the Middle Ages right up until the 1950s, a schizophrenic admitted to a psychiatric hospital usually had a very poor chance of ever coming out. Then came the first effective drugs to control psychotic episodes, known as the "phenothiazines," and even patients who had been on the back wards for years were able to regain enough control of their symptoms to be discharged. These drugs were first introduced in North America by a psychiatrist at McGill University in Montreal, and for about the last 36 years they have caused a revolution in how schizophrenics are treated, and how they are able to live. These medications, and the many antipsychotics or neuroleptics that have followed them, are certainly no cure, and often they do not even handle all the symptoms. However, they do provide control of the more intense manifestations, such as hallucinations, which would otherwise prevent schizophrenic people from functioning well in work or social relationships.

However these "wonder drugs" are not without side effects. Patients often complain that the drugs "zonk them out," and long-term use can result in spontaneous movements like tics, tremors and jerks that are difficult to control. Unlike normal facial expressions and gestures, these movements are not, however, directed at other people.

One form of tic is called "tardive dyskinesia," an abnormal behavior which develops slowly with prolonged use of the drugs, and involves uncontrollable movements of the mouth and tongue that can be decidedly unattractive and embarrassing. About 20 to 30% of schizophrenics taking neuroleptics for many years develop this condition, and in some, it cannot be reversed even if the drug is stopped. But people taking neuroleptics for illnesses other than schizophrenia are even more likely to get this side effect: virtually 100% develop these mouth movements if the drugs are taken long enough.

In contrast, about 3% of schizophrenic people develop this side effect each year that they take these drugs, and this percentage accumulates over the years. However, many people simply do not develop tardive dyskinesia at all. Research is urgently needed to find out what protects these people, since such knowledge could be used to defend others against this problem.

The neuroleptic drugs are important not only in treating schizophrenic episodes, but their continued use is very important to prevent a recurrence of these severe symptoms. Failure to continue to take these medications is a common cause of outbreaks of psychotic behavior.

There are many such drugs, each with its own effects, potency, side effects and risk factors. Tables 2.1 and 2.2 are excerpted from a recent handbook for psychiatrists and pharmacists showing some of the trade-offs involved with several of the most common neuroleptic medications. Notice the considerable variation in dosage and effects involved. As a result of these differences in potency and consequences, psychiatrists need to exercise very careful judgment in prescribing these medications.

Patients who fail to continue taking their appropriate medications can all too often go from talking to their hallucinations in a hospital ward, to arguing with them on a park bench. But long before such relapse problems surface it is likely that the schizophrenic's schooling, vocational training and development of social skills were interrupted by the disease, so he has difficulty getting work, and finds it hard to make friends. He may look, sound and act quite strange at times. His family may have become too discouraged to want to deal with him — they also have undergone a great deal of suffering.

Social skills training, appropriate housing and supervision, vocational rehabilitation, family education and support, and self-help groups for both families and the schizophrenics themselves may all be necessary before the victim of this disease can cope productively with life in the community. Programs to assist in developing social and other essential skills come in many forms, even including video tapes targeted at the patients themselves.

It turns out that many of these programs are more effective if they start in the hospital, rather than after discharge, and if there is a coordinated follow-up by various community agencies. While this approach tends to be more expensive, the results appear to be better than if the programs are begun after the patient leaves the hospital.

Table 2.1
Frequency of Adverse Reactions of Oral Neuroleptics

Reaction	Phenothiazines			Thioxan-	Butyro-	Diphenylbutyl-	Dibenzox-	Dihydro-
	Aliphatic	Piperazine	Piperidine	thenes	phenone	piperidine	azepine	indolone
Drowsiness, sedation	> 30%	2-10%	10-30%	10-30%	2-10%	10-30%	> 30%	> 30%
Extrapyramidal Effects								
Parkinsonism	10-30%	> 30%	2-10%	> 30%	> 30%	10-30%	> 30%	> 30%
Akathisia	2-10%	> 30%	2-10%	> 30%	> 30%	10-30%	> 30%	> 30%
Dystonic reactions	2-10%	10-30%	< 2%	10-30%	> 30%	10-30%	10-30%	> 30%
Cardiovascular Effects								
Orthostatic hypotension	> 30%	2-10%	10-30%	> 30%	2-10%	10-30%	10-30%	2-10%
Tachycardia	10-30%	2-10%	2-10%	2-10%	< 2%	2-10%	10-30%	< 2%
ECG abnormalities **	10-30%	2-10%	10-30%	2-10%	< 2%	2-10%	< 2%	< 2%
Cardiac arrhythmias	2-10%	-	10-30%	< 2%	< 2%	< 2%	-	-
Anticholinergic Effects	10-30%	2-10%	10-30%	10-30%	10-30%	10-30%	10-30%	10-30%
Endocrine Effects								
Inhibition of ejaculation	2-10%	2-10%	10-30%	< 2%	< 2%	-	2-10%	-
Weight gain	> 30%	2-10%	10-30%	10-30%	< 2%	2-10%	< 2%	< 2%
Skin Reactions								
Photosensitivity	2-10%	2-10%	2-10%	< 2%	< 2%	< 2%	< 2%	-
Rashes	2-10%	< 2%	10-30%	10-30%	< 2%	2-10%	2-10%	2-10%
Abnormal skin pigmentation	10-30%	< 2%	2-10%	< 2%	< 2%	-	-	-
Ocular Effects								
Lenticular pigmentation	2-10%	< 2%	2-10%	2-10%	< 2%	< 2%	< 2%	-
Pigmentary retinopathy	2-10%	< 2%	10-30%	-	-	-	-	-
Blood dyscrasias	2-10%	< 2%	2-10%	< 2%	< 2%	-	< 2%	< 2%
Cholestatic jaundice	< 2%	< 2%	< 2%	< 2%	< 2%	-	< 2%	< 2%
Cholestatic jaundice	< 2%	< 2%	< 2%	< 2%	< 2%	< 2%	< 2%	-
Epileptic seizures	2-10%	< 2%	< 2%	2-10%	< 2%	2-10%	< 2%	< 2%

Source: Bezchlibnyk-Butler, K. and Jeffries, J. (1990) *Clinical Handbook of Psychotropic Drugs.* Hogrefe & Huber Publishers: Toronto.

Table 2.2
A Comparison of Depot Neuroleptics

	Flupenthixol Decan. (Fluanxol)	Fluphenazine Enanthate (Moditen; Prolixin)	Fluphenazine Decanoate (Modecate; Prolixin)	Fluspirilene (Imap)	HaloperidolDecanoate (Haldol LA)	Pipotiazine Palmitate (Piportil L4)
Chemical Class	Thioxanthene	Piperazine pheno-thiazine	Piperazine pheno-thiazine	Diphenylbutyl-piperidine	Butyrophenone	Piperidine pheno-thiazine
Form	Esterified with a 10-carbon chain fatty acid and dissolved in vegetable oil. Must be hydrolyzed to free flupenthixol. Metabolites inactive.	Esterified with a 7-carbon chain fatty acid and dissolved in sesame oil. Must be hydrolyzed to free fluphenazine.	Esterified with a 10-carbon chain fatty acid and dissolved in sesame oil. Must be hydrolyzed to free fluphenazine.	Drug in a microcrystal-line form in an aqueous suspension. Immediately active on injection.Does not have to be hydro-lyzed.	Esterified with a 10-carbon chain fatty acid and dissolved in sesame oil. Must be hydrolyzed to free haloperidol.	Esterified with palmitic acid in sesame oil. Must be hydrolyzed to free to pipothiazine.
Strength supplied	2% - 20 mg/ml 10% - 100 mg/ml	25 mg/ml	25 mg/ml 100 mg/ml (investigational)	2 mg/ml 10 mg/ml	50 mg/ml 100 mg/ml	25 mg/ml 50 mg/ml
Usual dose range	20 - 80 mg	25 - 100 mg	12.5 - 50 mg	2 - 10 mg	50 - 300 mg	50 - 300 mg
Maximum dose in literature	800 mg/week	1250 mg/wk (Dencker)	400 mg/week (Clarke)	60 mg/week (Clarke)	1200 mg/injection (Chouinard)	600 mg/injection
Usual duration of action	3 weeks	2 weeks	4 weeks	1.5 weeks	4 weeks	4 weeks
Dose equivalency to 100 mg CPZ (approximate)	1.8 mg (50 mg q 4 wks)	0.93 mg/day (13 mg q 2 weeks)	0.46 mg/day (13 mg q 4 weeks)	0.3 mg/day (2 mg q 1 wk, females, 3 mg q 1 wk, males)	(1.1 mg/day) (30 mg q 4 wks)	0.85 mg/day (24 mg q 4 weeks)
PHARMACOKINETICS						
Onset of action	24 - 72 hours	24 - 96 hrs	Approx. 4 hrs	Within a few days	48 - 72 hrs	
Peak plasma level	4 - 7 days	2 - 5 days	Within a few hrs	Within 24 hrs	3 - 9 days	Approx. 4 days
Elimination half-life	8 days (after single injection) 17 days (multiple dosing)	3 1/2 - 4 days (after single injection)	6 - 10 days (single injection) 14.3 days (multiple dosing)	Approx. 9 days. Slowly excreted: less than 50% in 7 days, (approx. 70 % of drug excreted in 27 days)	18 - 21 days	6 - 11 days (rat), 8-9 days (dog). Approx. 10% of peak plasma drug level still detectable in plasma 45 days after an injection

Source: Bezchlibnyk-Butler, K. and Jeffries, J. (1990) *Clinical Handbook of Psychotropic Drugs.* Hogrefe & Huber Publishers: Toronto.

Families are able to cope much better once they understand the disease, learn how to deal with certain aspects of behavior, and know that they have many resources for support, advice and counseling. Self-help groups for families and friends have been formed all over the world. They provide direct support and guidance, develop recommendations for improved health care, and help raise funds for schizophrenia research.

While some individuals with this problem must undergo repeated admissions to various hospitals and cannot yet be helped very much, at the other end of the scale it is known that the disorder can arrest at any stage, and some people do recover. Fortunately, the old adage, "once a schizophrenic, always a schizophrenic" no longer holds. About 25% of people with a schizophrenic-like illness have only one episode and recover completely. Psychiatrists diagnose such people as having a "schizophreniform" illness. Recent studies suggest that 50% may recover quite completely by the time they reach 45-55 years of age.

Even people who have been merely surviving on hospital back wards for decades have been shown in several studies to be able to function in the community if they are given appropriate support and maintain a program of medication.

Actually there has been quite a major and interesting breakthrough recently in this area. A medication, commercially known as Clozaril, and whose generic name is clozapine, has been shown to have remarkable powers in helping those who have failed to respond to a long list of other anti-psychotic medications. The drug was first created in 1961, and introduced in Europe about 10 years later. A number of studies since then have shown that it does indeed have unique capabilities. Patients often respond strongly, and some actually become independent. In addition, the side effects are generally minimal, compared to other high powered medications aimed at schizophrenia. The medication was approved for use in the USA during February of 1990. In Canada its use is allowed with special governmental permission for each case. This drug has caused quite a stir, for several reasons.

One is that the drug itself has several problems. Most notably, it can kill people. Extensive studies have shown that a small percent of users are likely to develop "agranulocytosis" a disease which reduces one's ability to produce white blood cells, which are heavily involved in the body's defense against infection. A bit less than half of the patients who get this condition die from it, though the problem can be turned around by withdrawing use of clozapine.

Another problem is that not everyone can handle this particular medication. About 40% of the people who might in theory benefit from it either do not respond at all, or have such severe reactions that it's use has to be discontinued. Even those for whom it works effectively still require extensive psychotherapy, and training in social skills to help them function in places other than mental hospitals.

A third interesting element here is that it is expensive, with a cost of some $8,500 per year. The company which produces it, Sandoz, also requires that it not be sold in pharmacies, even with a prescription. Instead, to help monitor the risk with agranulocytosis, it is made available only in the context of a "Patient Management System," which has also caused quite a stir. This approach requires that patients be given regular medical exams and blood tests, and Sandoz has contracted with specific firms such that only they will be allowed to take weekly blood samples and test them for white blood cells.

This is definitely a unique approach to the selling of drugs. As a result the firm is under strong pressure to reduce the price. It turns out that in Oklahoma if it were used on all eligible patients the cost would exceed the state's entire mental health budget. In addition, in parts of Europe that drug is available for prices in the neighborhood of $1,500 per year.

But the firm explains that these lower prices reflect different regulatory cost, and various forms of price controls, and that in the USA the goal is to produce the highest possible level of patient safety. It is agreed by many that if a number of deaths did occur due to the drug it would likely be withdrawn from the market, and in this situation thousands, perhaps hundreds of thousands of schizophrenics would be denied the benefits which the medication appears able to produce. Meanwhile the various regulatory agencies are deciding what to do. Some critics note that while Medicaid is willing to pay very large amounts per year to keep

Figure 2.4
Patient Management System for Clozaril

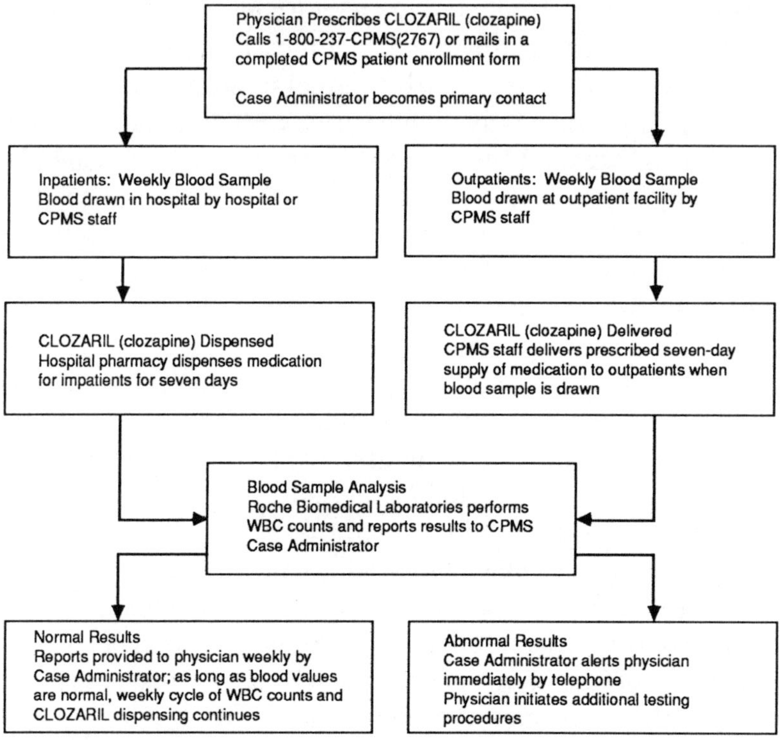

people alive, upwards of $50,000 for kidney dialysis for example, it seems inappropriate to make such a big commotion about $8,700 to dramatically help a very large number of schizophrenics.

In any case there is a logical problem here. If the patients are improved enough to return to work, they would become no longer eligible for Medicaid, which provides the money for the medication which helps them be able to hold a job. Nonetheless, the experience with this drug is very helpful in many ways, and the reality that it can be highly effective for certain people is most encouraging, and may lead to the development of related drugs which are less expensive and perhaps have fewer potentially difficult side effects.

In addition to the various technical treatment solutions which psychiatrists and other scientists have come up with it is important to mention what may seem like a more human side of this world. Available to schizophrenics, as well as others suffering from a variety of mental illnesses are a wide range of privately supported residential treatment facilities throughout the USA. These are generally expensive by normal standards, and the public sector funding which is available varies with the state or province where one is located. Therefore private insurance is often involved as a third party to help pay for the use of these facilities. These treatment centers, whether public or private, are an important aspect of many mental health disorders, since the problems are often more difficult than can be handled by immediate family and friends.

While these centers vary, they are all oriented toward comfort, care, therapy, and rehabilitation. Some are modest operations located in a large house, while others are extensive hospitals, sometimes located in very attractive settings. Without intending to single out any one of these operations for special scrutiny, it is worthwhile to briefly look at a few to get some sense of this specialized world. The first two figures below are from a brochure describing one smaller scale center, which deals exclusively with schizophrenic patients, and is located in Georgia. This facility utilizes an intensive treatment approach, works closely with local medical schools, and has published studies showing a high one year post-release success rate. The general cost is about $3,400 per month, including housing.

A second example below is taken from a private 150 bed treatment center in New England. To illustrate the variation in these rehabilitation facilities, this one is non-profit and over 150 years old. It also includes an extensive dairy farm, which helps finance the treatment programs involved. This center has a wide variety of drug and other mental health related programs.

Some experts feel that private treatment centers can be excessively expensive, as they can cost upwards of $700 per day and in addition some have not regularly demonstrated greatly superior results. But they have become popular, and often teach coping techniques which can be repeatedly utilized long after the

Figure 2.5
Illustration of A Smaller Treatment Center in Georgia

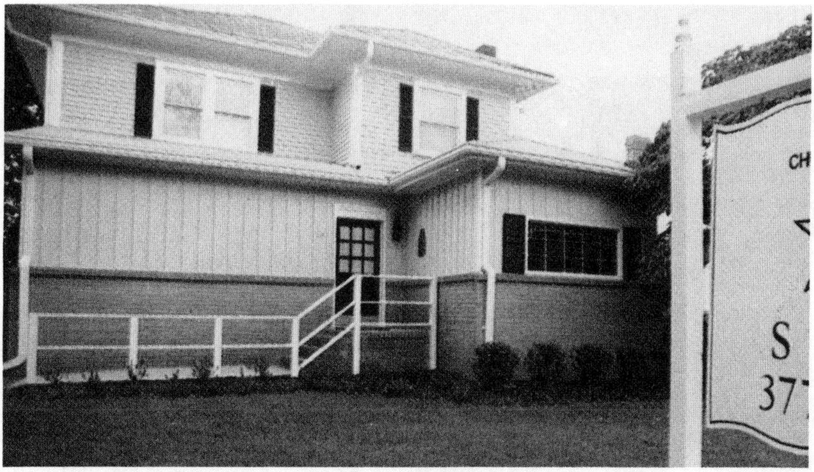

Figure 2.6
Counseling Session at a Smaller Treatment Center

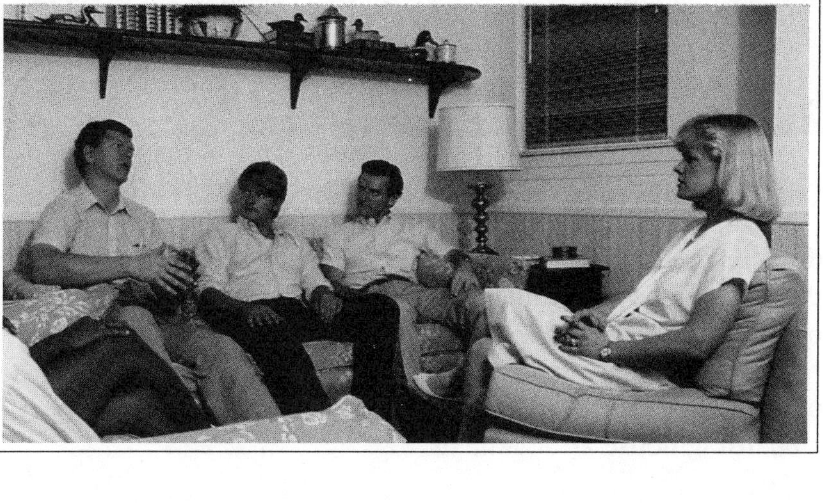

Figure 2.7
Overview of the Recreation Center at a Private Non-Profit Treatment Center in New England

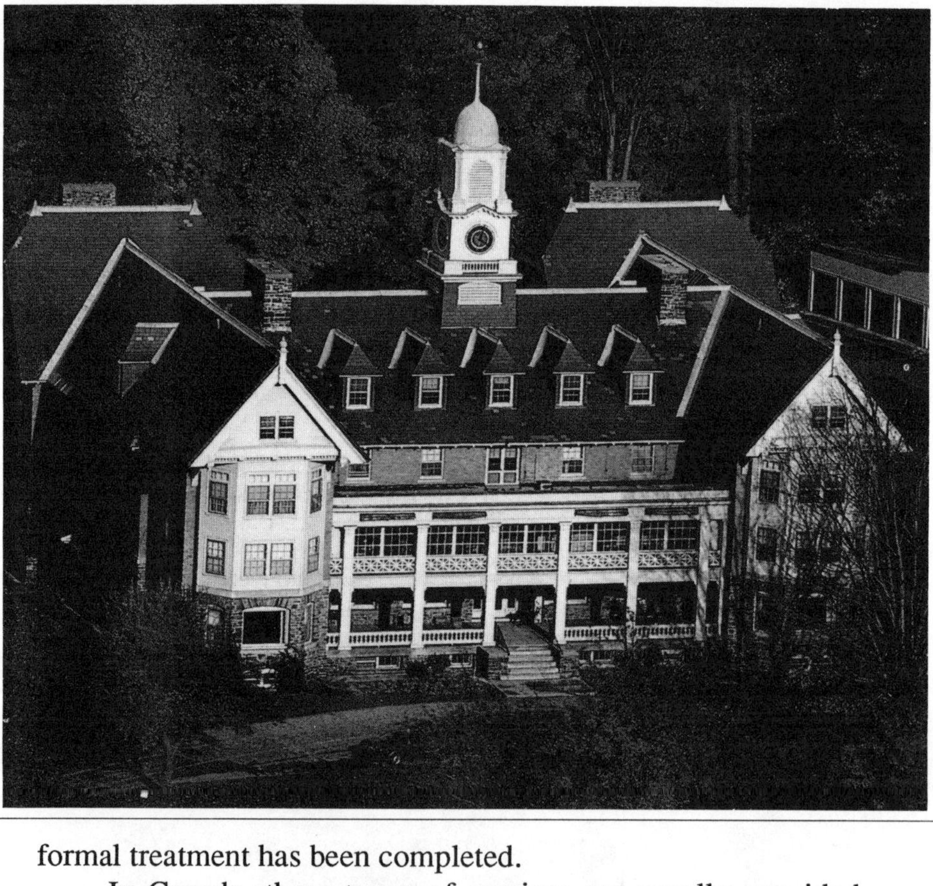

formal treatment has been completed.

In Canada, these types of services are usually provided directly by the government supported health care system. After the patient recovers from the psychosis in a provincial psychiatric or general hospital, the rehabilitation is usually carried out in programs that are available in the patient's community, while he or she lives at home, in an apartment, or perhaps in some from of a boarding house arrangement.

*** Research

There is now a great need for carefully controlled studies to determine which combinations of treatments, patient characteristics, and stage of the illness give the best results. If we were able to determine this optimal mix, the benefits would be spectacular, to the patients, families, and the community.

Further investigation of the dopamine receptor system mentioned earlier not only promises to unravel some biochemical mechanisms underlying the disease, but also to yield better drug therapy. Some medications now used to control symptoms appear to do so by occupying those receptors, so that excessive amounts of dopamine cannot attach to them.

Fortunately, we now have available a number of quite powerful and interesting computerized techniques for learning about the brain's physical anatomy, and remarkably, also how it actually is functioning. In the past such studies were largely done via autopsies of victims of various diseases. But these new techniques are helping to improve the understanding of the mental illnesses, and how to deal with them. Let's take a quick look at some of this technology, because it is important, and certain to become more so in the near future.

Many people have heard of a "CAT scan." This is a device aimed at understanding the anatomy of the brain, or other body systems. The initials stand for Computerized Axial Tomography. This technique uses the computer to analyze many cross sectional "slices" (tomo is from a Greek word roughly meaning slice), taken at different axes or angles of view. In this approach, a low powered X-ray beam is sent through the patient's head, and a sophisticated machine measures how much radiation actually penetrates the structure being analyzed. The interesting element here is that these X-rays are sent in from many different angles, or axes, thus making it possible to come up with a cross-section picture of the brain, from any angle desired.

Another approach is called MRI, for Magnetic Resonance Imaging. When tissues are placed in a magnetic field, and then subjected to certain radio frequencies, the tissues themselves emit a signal which can actually be measured. In practice many thousands of such signals are generated, and the computer puts them together into a two-dimensional picture of the brain, or whatever system is being investigated. It is generally agreed that MRI produces a better picture than CAT. However MRI machines can cost $1.5 million, quite expensive, which has given rise to certain short cut methods, which produce results almost as good, but at less cost. Figure 2.8 shows a more or less typical main component of an MRI system. Figures 2.9 and 2.10 illustrate the sorts of pictures which are generated by the MRI system.

Figure 2.8
Magnetic Resonance Imaging Equipment

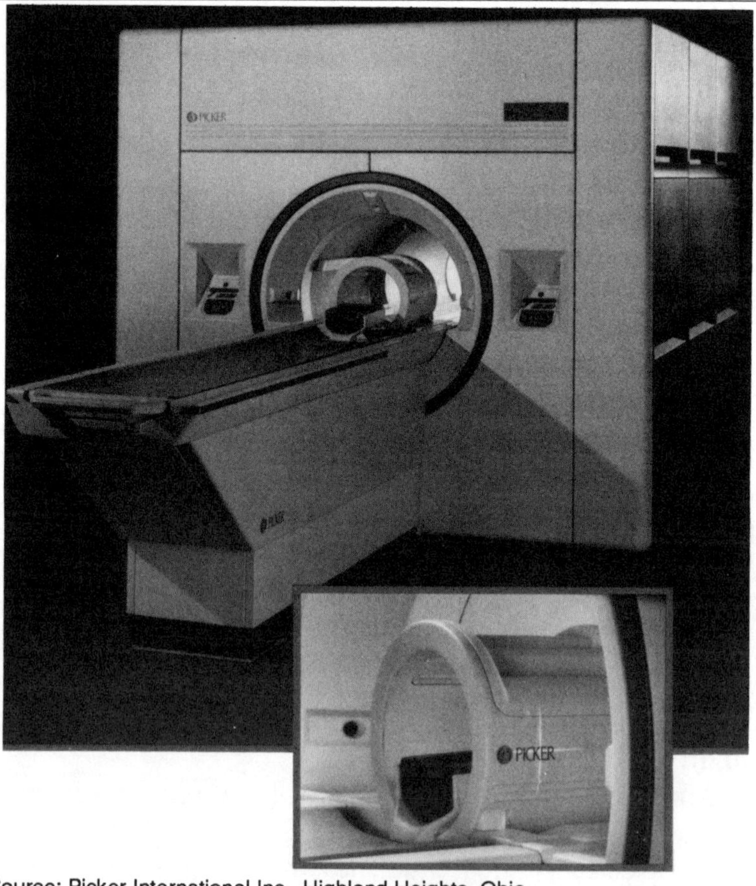

Source: Picker International Inc., Highland Heights, Ohio.

Figure 2.9
Example of MRI Generated Results

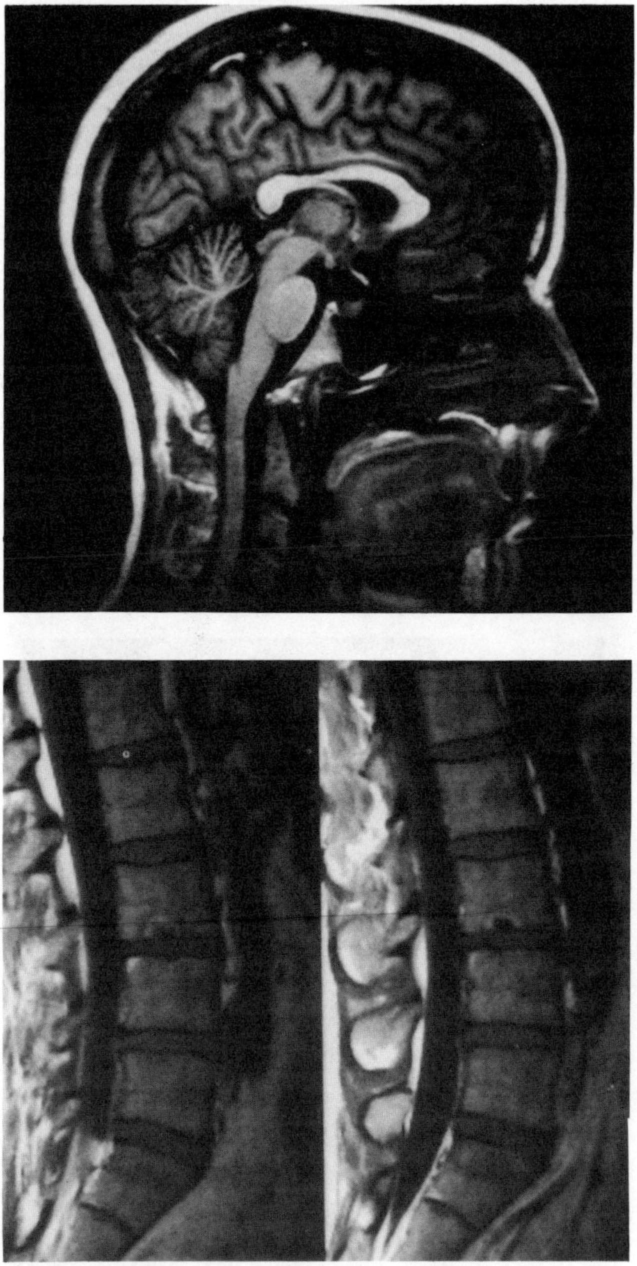

Source: Picker International Inc., Highland Heights, Ohio.

Figure 2.10
Further Example of MRI Pictures

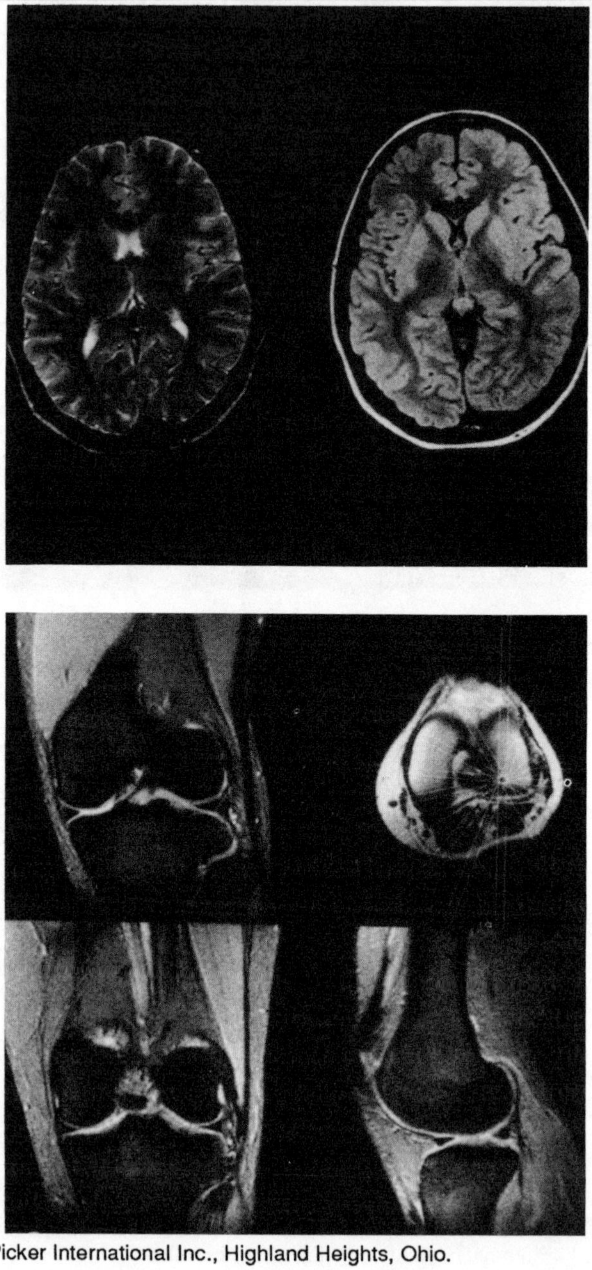

Source: Picker International Inc., Highland Heights, Ohio.

In using these various anatomy oriented techniques, psychiatrists have discovered that many people with schizophrenia have physical changes in their brains, compared to normals. In particular, the ventricle areas, where cerebrospinal fluid circulates appear to be enlarged, but it is not known for sure yet if this condition causes, or is caused by schizophrenia.

In contrast to CAT and MRI, Positron Emission Tomography (PET) scans can provide pictures of how the brain is actually functioning, rather than "merely" its anatomy. An example of such equipment is shown in Figure 2.11. Very small and harmless

Figure 2.11
Illustrative PET Scan Machine

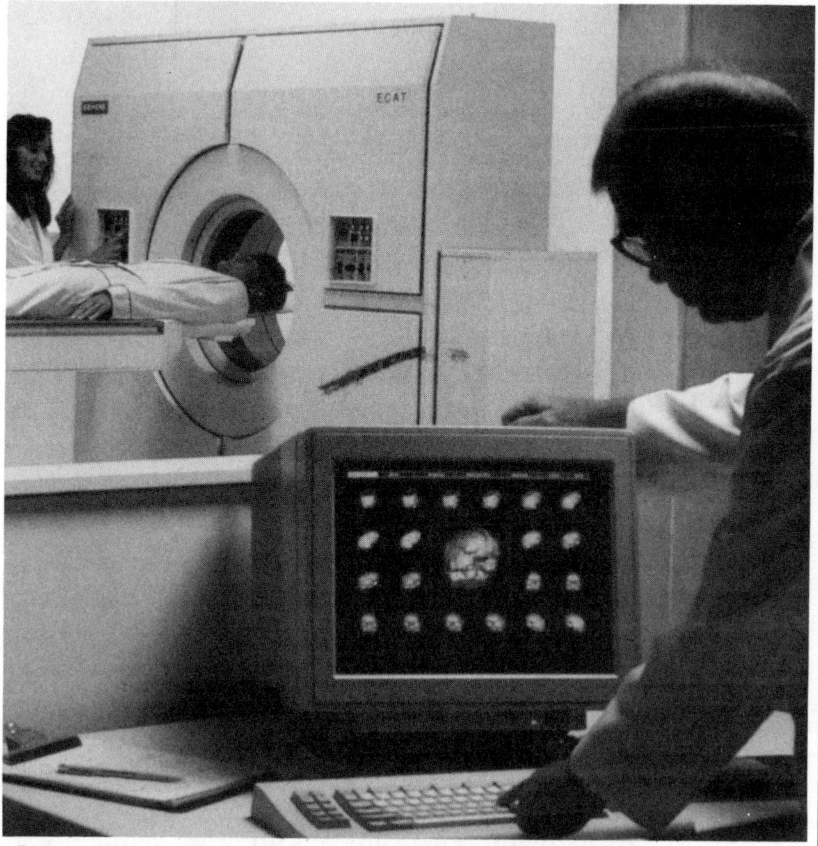

Source: Siemens Medical Systems, Inc., Hoffman Estates, Illinois.

amounts of radioactive material can be added to injections of glucose, the brain's main fuel, or to a natural substance which becomes dopamine when injected into the bloodstream, or even to drugs used to treat schizophrenia. The radioactivity allows these materials to be seen on the scan as they accumulate in various parts of the brain. The PET machine acts somewhat like an extremely sophisticated Geiger counter, measuring the very small amounts of radioactivity in the glucose circulating through the brain. This approach is not similar to an X-ray machine, which actually emits radioactivity itself.

The patient lies on a stretcher with his head in the scanner, and pictures emerge showing if various parts of the brain are using glucose normally, whether there are abnormal levels of dopamine in some areas, or how well a drug is blocking dopamine receptors.

With this technique, scientists can now see how much of a certain drug is needed to eliminate symptoms, and early studies indicate that the dosages required may be considerably less than was previously believed necessary. This new understanding could go a long way toward reducing or eliminating side effects, and in tailoring dosages to the individual. However, it will take a few years of research to put this knowledge into practice.

In the next few decades, advances in genetics may unearth the underlying physical causes of many mental illnesses. For example, a massive project is currently underway to characterize the human genome, the complete set of instructions for making a human being that are written in the DNA (deoxyribonucleic acid) found in the 46 chromosomes that every human cell contains.

In the 35 years since James Watson and Francis Crick discovered the complex structure of DNA, only a tiny fraction of its instructions have been deciphered. New techniques are available now that are speeding up these investigations.

Each chromosome has thousands of locations on it called genes, and each gene contains blueprints to regulate certain cells. Finding one gene that has a defect associated with a certain disease is a needle-in-a-haystack operation, but such a discovery would open the way to pinpointing where the abnormality lies in the gene — where one of its many blueprints has an error that is giving improper instructions to some cells. This is no small task — it is perhaps the equivalent of finding a few typographical errors in an entire encyclopedia.

Pinpointing a defective gene for schizophrenia would be an enormous breakthrough. It would make possible the construction of a test which could be administered in the early stage of pregnancy to detect which babies might be at risk for the disease. However, this sort of capability is still a long way off. Preliminary work in several countries studying various schizophrenic members of the same family indicate that there are probably many different kinds of schizophrenia: some genetic, some not, or indeed several different genetic variations of the disorder.

The ultimate goal is gene replacement therapy, where a normal gene would be attached to an organism that would take it into the cell to replace an abnormal gene, but this approach is even more years away than a prenatal test.

Further research is also needed into the interesting gender differences involved with schizophrenia. The average age for the hospitalization of females with this disorder is 25, compared to only 18 for men. Women also tend to have more success in overcoming it – and they have lower rates of suicide, unemployment, hospitalization and disruptive relationships.

Some of the possibilities being explored in the studies of these disparities are brain differences between the sexes, hormonal influence, and social factors. For example, estrogen hormones tend to block the action of dopamine, and of course women have far more estrogen than men. The later onset of the disease in women may also give them more time to complete their education and develop work and social skills so that they are better able to cope with the onset of the problem once it does develop.

*** *For Further Information*

Organizations

Canadian Friends of Schizophrenics, #309, 95 Barber Greene Road, Don Mills, Ontario, M3C 3E9. Tel: (416) 445-8204, a support group for schizophrenics and their families. Chapters exist in many communities.

The National Alliance for the Mentally Ill. 2101 Wilson Boulevard, Suite 302, Arlington, VA 22201. (703) 524-7600.

Books

Bernheim, K.F., Levine R.R.J., and Beale, C.T. (1982). *The Caring Family.* New York: Random House.

Bezchlibnyk-Butler, K. and Jeffries, J. (1990). *Clinical Handbook of Psychotropic Drugs.* Toronto: Hogrefe & Huber Publishers.

Seeman, M.V., Littman, S.K., Plummer, E, Thornton, J.F. and Jeffries, J.J. (1982). *Living and Working with Schizophrenia.* Toronto: University of Toronto Press.

Thornton, John MD. (1991). *Schizophrenia Simplified, A Field Guide to the Social, Medical and Legal Complexities.* Toronto: Hogrefe & Huber Publishers. This is very practical spiral bound manual featuring a series of unique flow charts spelling out consequences of the disorder with respect to many important dimensions of interest to patients, but also to family members.

Torrey, E.F. (1983). *Surviving Schizophrenia, A Family Manual.* New York: Harper and Row.

Video Tapes

Liberman, R. (1989). *Social and Independent Living Skills.* A set of four video tapes of very high quality developed at UCLA to teach social adaptation, and to foster rehabilitation for disabled mental patients with serious mental disorders. These modules are widely used in both in- and outpatient settings, residential care facilities, private practice clinics, and community mental health centers. Available from Hogrefe & Huber Publishers, Toronto.

Chapter 3

Depression

Everyone has days when it feels like the entire earth is painted grey. We usually call this feeling depressed, and happily, such an outlook usually goes away in a relatively short time, especially when the sun comes out.

Not so with the group of illnesses that psychiatrists define as depressions. These are longer, more serious conditions that bring changes in mood, behavior and thinking, often along with severe physical symptoms, which do not lift with the unexpected arrival of a gift of flowers, or when friends encourage one to "snap out of it."

There is both a good and bad news element with this disorder. While it is one of the most common of all mental illnesses, but nonetheless about 90% of the people who develop this problem can be effectively treated.

About 1 in 4 women in North America are expected to become clinically depressed at some point in their lives. For men the figure is roughly 1 in 10. In most people these episodes are relatively shorted lived, lasting perhaps a year. But for about 30% of the victims, chronic depression sets in, and maintaining a normal life becomes impossible. Another troubling aspect about this problem is evidence showing that about 50% of the people who have had this disorder will at some point have another experience with it some years later.

Contrary to common impressions, clinical depression can develop at any age, and especially with regard to young people this disorder is widely suspected to be a major factor in suicide, which is the third most common cause of death for people aged 15 to 24.

In general, compared to adults, children tend to express this disorder differently, especially in the elementary school years. A child who is usually lively may become irritable and poorly behaved without any evident reason. A preschool child, in contrast, may become unduly quiet, withdrawn and unhappy. In adolescence, many teenagers will complain of feeling helpless and unworthy. Both children and adolescents with this problem may have sleep disturbances, such as an unwillingness to go to sleep, and frequent or early waking.

Strictly speaking, there are two main types of depression, technically called "affective disorders." Major depressive or unipolar disorder is very common indeed: up to 20 percent of North Americans will have it at some time in their lives. It is well known that women seek help for it twice as often as men, but that does not necessarily mean it is twice as common in them. Statistically, women are more likely to seek professional help for all sorts of medical problems.

For weeks the person with depression may have had trouble eating and sleeping, his appetite is gone, he's losing weight, and is wide awake at 5 a.m. Normal activities have lost their appeal. The victim of this disorder cannot get enthusiastic about anything, and dithers instead of making decisions. Everything seems negative. The future looks as dismal as the present, everything has gone wrong and it is strictly the fault of the depressed person. Feelings of worthlessness are almost overwhelming, and suicide is often a recurrent thought.

The other major type of affective disorder disease is called manic-depression, and is referred to as bipolar, because its two phases are very distinct. In the manic phase, the person is on a real high, usually hyperactive and feeling unbeatable, and not all these people are teenage males. Unfortunately, those with this disorder may be also extremely irritable and can show a devastating lack of judgment — telling a boss where he can go, surprising, and dismaying, a spouse by wiping out their bank account with a mink coat and a grand piano that no one can play. But, when one hits the other extreme, severe symptoms of depression often result.

Between these two extremes there are normal periods that can last for months or years — there are wide variations among individuals. Some people suffering from this disease have many more periods of mania than depression, and vice versa.

Jack, for example, at 36 years of age, was a successful real estate salesman whose family noticed he was working harder than usual, and seemed to have boundless energy. He seemed to need only a few hours of sleep, he wanted sex with his wife more often, and he began to talk about pulling off extraordinary deals. When his family and friends argued these deals didn't seem realistic, he got insulted and accused them of not having confidence in his abilities. But when he talked about buying the Peace Bridge across the Niagara River near his home, they knew there was something definitely wrong.

He steadfastly refused to see a doctor, but late one night he was stopped by police for speeding, and became abusive when the officer wanted a breathalyzer test. When he phoned his lawyer from the police station, the lawyer convinced the police to take him to a hospital. The examining doctor didn't think he was an imminent danger to himself or others, the grounds on which he could have been admitted against his will, but when the officer pointed out he had been driving at 90 mph, the doctor completed a form to compel Jack to remain under examination for 72 hours. In the hospital, Jack continued to brag about his feats as a salesman, talking rapidly and sometimes incoherently, and sleeping very little. He was given a sedating drug, Clonazepam, and began taking lithium. Within two weeks he had settled down considerably and was able to understand what he had been doing, although he was extremely ashamed of it. In another week, he was able to return home and to his work, and his family relations returned to the level they had been at before the manic episode. He did not continue to try to buy the Peace Bridge.

Besides these two major depressive disorders, there are several less common variations. In recent years, one has been dubbed "seasonal affective disorder" or SAD, because it appears to come in the fall and end in spring. There's still some controversy about this one, such as whether the seasonal pattern remains, or it subsequently reappears at other times of the year in the same person. Another variety is called somatizing depression, from the Greek word for body, where physical complaints predominate, but no cause for them can be found. It does not have the same conspicuous mood symptoms, but the person is generally weighted down by a continuous pattern of gloomy thoughts. Still another variant is a chronic low level depression with fewer physical symptoms, but an inability to feel happy or get any pleasure out of life.

*** Causes

There is considerable scientific evidence that some distinct groups of people seem more susceptible to depression than others. There certainly appears to be a genetic factor involved. Children in families where both parents have a clear affective disorder have a 30 to 40 percent likelihood of developing one as well. If one identical twin has a major depression, there is a 70 percent chance the other one will develop it. But in fraternal twins, the likelihood is only 25 percent.

Other psychiatric conditions, such as schizophrenia or agoraphobia, which is a great fear of open spaces, may bring a higher risk of depression, as the person becomes aware of declining capabilities or an inability to keep control over his own life.

Depression is fairly common in some clearly medical conditions such as hypothyroidism, where the thyroid gland is underactive, or in Cushing's disease, which involves the pituitary and adrenal glands.

Depression may be directly caused by a physical problem — a stroke may affect the part of the brain that controls mood, or kidney failure may cause a massive chemical imbalance. It may also be a reaction to the effect of various diseases on the sufferer's life.

This disorder is also a relatively common side effect of some drugs, including anti-hypertensives to reduce blood pressure, some beta-blockers used for heart disease and angina, and alcohol. In addition, the abuse of alcohol is often a cause of the disease. Such depressions may hang on and require treatment even after use of the drug in question has been stopped.

Major losses in childhood, such as the death of a parent, are more often found in the backgrounds of the depressed, but on the other hand, many people with these emotional traumas do not develop depression. There are protective factors against later depression, such as the resumption of stable and long-lasting family relationships. It may be the number or duration of adverse factors that makes the difference.

A study in a low-income housing area of London, for example, found that women were at highest risk of depression if they had lost a parent before they were 11 years old, they had three or more children under 14 living at home, they did not have a job outside the home, and they did not have someone close in whom they could confide.

Depression is found in all age groups, but the elderly are particularly susceptible, probably because they have many risk factors, such as physical illness and loss of those close to them, and often a great deal of loneliness.

*** Treatment

Due to the advances made by psychiatrists and other scientists over the last 20 years, depression is widely regarded as one of the major success stories for the field of psychiatry. Fortunately, our ability to prevent or treat this disorder has grown enormously, largely due to the development of better medications.

In general, the treatment of depression falls into three categories:

- biological
- psychological
- social

Biological Methods

The first of these broad approaches includes both anti-depressant drugs and electroconvulsive therapy (ECT) or "shock" treatment.

Interestingly, despite the "emotional" connection implied with this disease, two different biochemical systems of neurotransmitters have been heavily implicated as causes of depression. These are the chemicals essential to the transmission of electrical impulses from one nerve cell to another. Drugs that are effective in dealing with depression have shown that the two neurotransmitters involved are serotonin and noradrenaline.

In general there are today more than 20 anti-depressants from which psychiatrists can choose to treat this disorder. The main class of effective drugs are called "tricyclic anti-depressants" or TCAs, developed in the 1950s. They block the reabsorption of neurotransmitters after they have been released into the gap that separates nerve cells. The result is an accumulation of these substances to make up for the low level of them that may be present in depression.

Many of these medications have side effects, but they are not usually damaging: dry mouth, and a slight blurring of vision, both of which tend to improve over time. Another common problem is a slight reduction in blood pressure that may cause light-headedness if someone stands up quickly from a lying position. Table 3.1 is an excerpt from a handbook regarding psychotropic medications, and this section illustrates some of the side effects, and how often they might occur, comparing some of the various drugs used for depression.

Another class of drugs used in treating depression are called "monoamineoxidase inhibitors" (MAOIs), and their value in depression was discovered accidentally. These were previously employed to treat tuberculosis, but after a while it was clearly observed that TB patients who were also depressed became much less so when using them.

MAO is a substance normally used in the breakdown of norepinephrine and serotonin, and reducing its effectiveness increases the amount of the two neurotransmitters available. The end result is the same as with the TCAs, but the MAOIs are trickier

Table 3.1
Frequency of Adverse Reactions — Antidepressants

Reaction	Amoxapine	Maprotiline	Trazodone	Isocarboxazid	Phenelzine	Tranylcypromine	Bupropion [1]	Fluoxetine
Anticholinergic Effects								
Dry mouth	> 30%	> 30%	2-10%	10-30%	> 30%	10-30%	10-30%	2-10%
Blurred vision	2-10%	10-30%	2-10%	2-10%	10-30%	2-10%	2-10%	2-10%
Constipation	> 30%	10-30%	2-10%	2-10%	10-30%	2-10%	2-10%	2-10%
Sweating	2-10%	2-10%	-	< 2%	2-10%	-	2-10%	2-10%
Delayed micturition*	10-30%	2-10%	< 2%	2-10%	2-10%	2-10%	2-10%	< 2%
CNS Effects								
Drowsiness, sedation	10-30%	10-30%	10-30%	2-10%	10-30%	10-30%	2-10%	10-30%
Insomnia	10-30%	< 2%	< 2%	2-10%	10-30%	10-30%	2-10%	10-30%
Excitement/Hypomania***	2-10%	2-10%	-	2-10%	10-30%	10-30%	2-10%	10-30%
Disorientation/Confusion	2-10%	2-10%	< 2%	2-10%	2-10%	2-10%	2-10%	10-30%
Headache	2-10%	< 2%	2-10%	10-30%	2-10%	-	2-10%	10-30%
Extrapyramidal Effects								
Unspecified	2-10%	2-10%	2-10%	2-10%	2-10%	< 2%	2-10%	2-10%
Tremor (Fine)	2-10%	10-30%	2-10%	2-10%	10-30%	2-10%	2-10%	10-30%
Cardiovascular Effects								
Orthostatic hypotension/ dizziness	10-30%	2-10%	10-30%	10-30%	10-30%	10-30%	2-10%	10-30%
Tachycardia	10-30%	2-10%	2-10%	-	10-30%	10-30%	< 2%	-
ECG changes**	< 2%	< 2%	< 2%	-	-	-	< 2%	< 2%
Cardiac arrhythmia	< 2%	< 2%	< 2%	2-10%	-	< 2%	< 2%	< 2%
G.I. distress (nausea)	2-10%	2-10%	10-30%	10-30%	10-30%	2-10%	2-10%	10-30%
Dermatitis, rash	10-30%	10-30%	< 2%	2-10%	< 2%	2-10%	2-10%	2-10%
Weakness, fatigue	2-10%	-	< 2%	2-10%	< 2%	<2%	2-10%	-
Weight gain (over 6 kg)	< 2%	10-30%	2-10%	10-30%	10-30%	2-10%	< 2%	-
Sexual disturbances	2-10%	< 2%	< 2%	2-10%	10-30%	2-10%	< 2%	2-10%
Epileptic seizures [c]	< 2%	2-10%	< 2%	-	< 2%	-	< 2%	< 2%

Source: Bezchlibnyk-Butler, K. and Jeffries, J. (1990) *Clinical Handbook of Psychotropic Drugs.* Hogrefe & Huber Publishers: Toronto.

to use. If the patient's diet contains high amounts of tyramine, found in wine, cheese and other foods, the result can be potentially dangerous high blood pressure. People taking MAOIs need careful guidance by a nutritionist. Partly due to these difficulties, MAOIs are used less often than the tricyclics, but, for some people, they are the only thing that works.

For the manic-depressive in the acute phase of mania, major tranquillizers are usually required to reduce the hyperactivity and bring mood and behavior back to a normal level. When there are recurrent swings from depression to mania and back again, periodically disrupting the continuity of a person's life, lithium may be effective as a preventative, to reduce the risk of relapse. It may need to be continued for extended periods of time, with regular tests to check that the appropriate drug levels are in the blood.

For those in whom lithium is not effective, sometimes another medication, such as carbamazepine may be useful.

Of course any discussion of the modern medicinal treatment of depression needs to mention what some observers regard as the most promising of all the new drugs, one called fluoxetine, whose trade name is Prozac, produced by the Lilly company. This compound appears to have at least two strong advantages, which cause some people to regard it as a virtual wonder drug. First, it is at least as effective as other drugs in helping those with depression overcome their disorders. Second, it has apparently far fewer side effects, making it much easier to take, and to continue utilizing over long periods. Interestingly, this particular drug is not directly related to the tricyclics, nor the MAOIs, but represents something of a new path in the search for effective medications in this field.

Based on quite extensive data, it does appear that the use of this drug causes fewer complaints than either tricyclics, or MAOIs, as suggested by Table 3.2 which presents summary data and comments taken from a study of 2,938 subjects performed by Glenn L. Cooper and reported in the 1988 volume of the *British Journal of Psychiatry*.

Part of this article also presented several interesting graphs which nicely pull together some of the details which lie behind this summary. To provide a bit of the flavor of this area of high-

Table 3.2
Summary Quote from *British Journal of Psychiatry* 1988

Author:
Glen L. Cooper
Journal:
Br. J. Psychiatry 1988; 153 (suppl 3):77-86

- **Study Population**
  Data pooled from comparative clinical trials of 4,336 patients (primarily adults) with a major depressive disorder

Drug	No. of Patients	Dosage
Fluoxetine	N = 2,938	20-80 mg/day
Tricyclics (amitriptyline, imipramine, doxepin)	N = 599	Dose titrated
Placebo	N = 799	—

- **Study Design:**
  Most common design was a six-week, comparative, double-blind phase, followed by unblinded long-term treatment.

Adverse events

- **Incidence of Common TCA-Associated Side Effects**
  "Fluoxetine-treated patients had a higher incidence of nervousness, insomnia, and anxiety than patients on comparison drug or placebo, but for most patients these symptoms were mild and tolerable. In contrast, drowsiness was reported more frequently with TCAs than with fluoxetine."

"A sensitive indicator of the severity of an adverse event is the proportion of patients who discontinue [treatment]. ...nervousness, insomnia, and anxiety were infrequent reasons for discontinuation of fluoxetine. Discontinuations due to drowsiness and anticholinergic side-effects were greater with TCAs than with fluoxetine or placebo."

"The incidence of anticholinergic complaints was similar for fluoxetine- and placebo-treated patients."

Figure 3.1
The Most Common Adverse Events Associated with Discontinuation in Comparative Clinical Trials

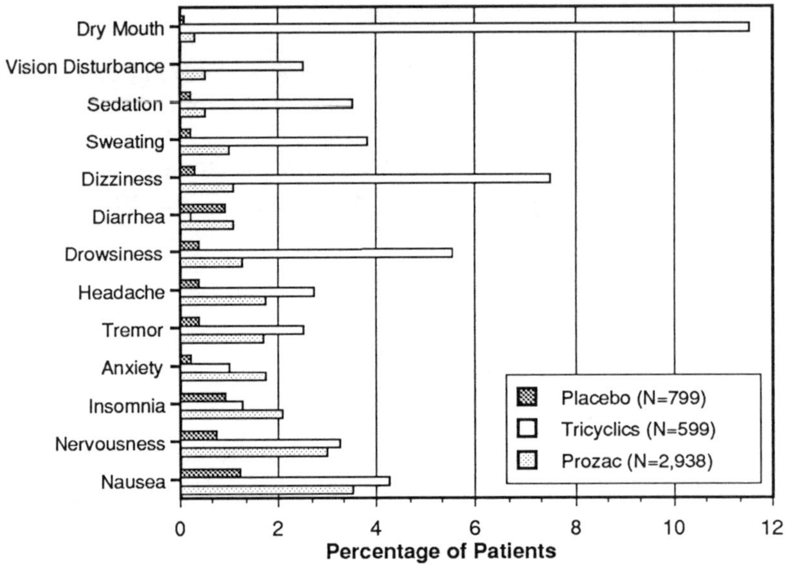

Source: Br. J. Psychiatry 1988; 153 (suppl 3):77-86

powered drug research, three of these charts are worth considering here. The first shows the most frequent causes of why people in the study discontinued taking their medication. As you know, the placebo group reported here concerns those subjects who were led to believe that they were being given an active medication, yet were really taking a completely inert pill.

Figure 3.2 shows the precentage of patients who experienced various "adverse events" while taking this drug, compared to those getting the fake pill, and those being given tricyclics as part of the study.

Another interesting graph from this study helps support the viewpoint that this particular medication is relatively safe for older patients as well, shown in Figure 3.3.

Figure 3.2
The Most Common Adverse Events with Fluoxetine in Comparative Clinical Trials

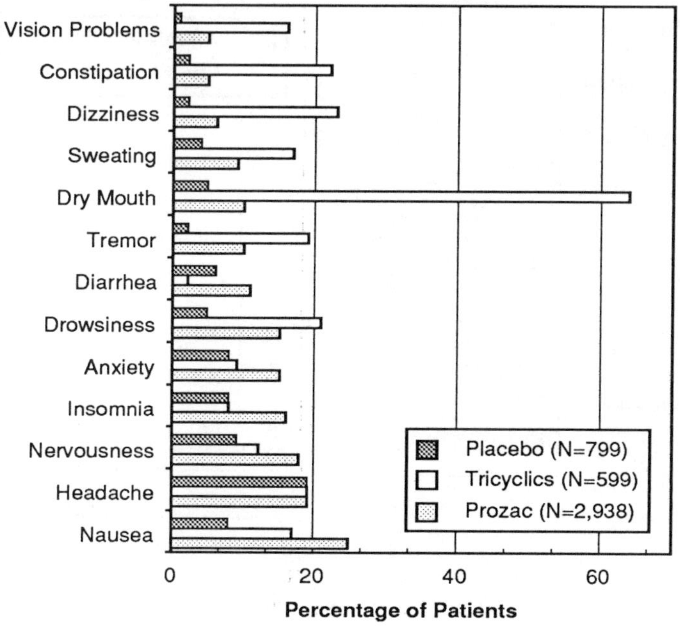

Source: Br. J. Psychiatry 1988; 153 (suppl 3):77-86

Readers with an interest in medical science per se might find the following excerpt from a brochure for physicians of considerable interest, as shown in Table 3.3. It nicely illustrates the language used to describe state-of-the-art results, and uncertainties, regarding a new and important medication. The specific findings reported are also quite interesting in their own right.

Without getting too scientific here, it is interesting to point out that the well known compound "tryptophan," which is available in a normal diet, is transformed by the body into a chemical messenger called "5-hydroxy-tryptophan," otherwise known as 5HT. As shown in Figure 3.4 below, it turns out that Fluoxetine acts like something of a substitute for 5HT, which is often found to be in low supply in people with depression. Another important

Figure 3.3
Adverse Events in Geriatric Patients vs All Patients Treated with Fluoxetine

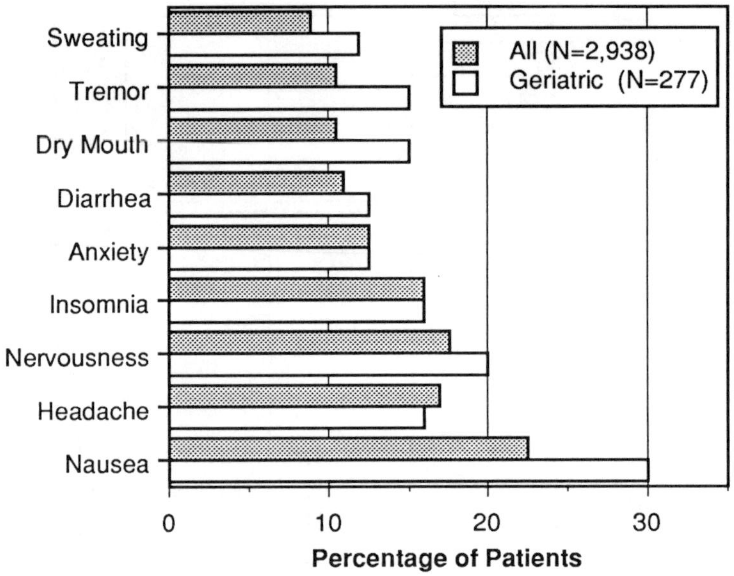

Source: Br. J. Psychiatry 1988; 153 (suppl 3):77-86

drug shown here, called "Reserpine," can interfere with the storage of 5HT in certain storage granules, which in turn can lead to a depletion of 5HT, which can lead to depression. But so can a diet low in tryptophan, although normal diets are not generally deficient in this area.

Another interesting drug addressed in this illustration is "amitriptyline," which retards the reabsorption of 5HT after it has been released from the cell body, and thus allows a larger amount of it to activate the neighboring cell. It is an effective antidepressant drug. Somewhat along this same line of reasoning, the so-called MAOI drugs (monoamine oxidase inhibitors), slow down the breakdown of 5HT into something called 5HIAA, and thus leave more 5HT available to relieve depression. Again, Fluoxetine acts like a substitute for 5HT, the general lack of which appears to be related to depression.

Table 3.3
Excerpt from Physician Pamphlet Regarding Clinical Pharmacology of Prozac

Pharmacodynamics

The antidepressant action of fluoxetine is presumed to be linked to its inhibition of CNS neuronal uptake of serotonin. Studies at clinically relevant doses in man have demonstrated that fluoxetine blocked the uptake of serotonin into human platelets. Studies in animals also suggest that fluoxetine is a much more potent uptake inhibitor of serotonin than of norepinephrine.

Antagonism of muscarinic, histaminergic, and α_1-adrenergic receptors has been hypothesized to be associated with various anticholinergic, sedative, and cardiovascular effects of classical tricyclic antidepressant drugs. Fluoxetine binds to these and other membrane receptors from brain tissue much less potently in vitro than do the tricyclic drugs.

Absorption, Distribution, Metabolism, and Excretion

Systemic Bioavailability — in man, following a single oral 40-mg dose, peak plasma concentrations of fluoxetine from 15 to 55 ng/mL are observed after six to eight hours.

Food does not appear to affect the systemic bioavailability of fluoxetine, although it may delay its absorption inconsequentially. Thus, fluoxetine may be administered with or without food.

Protein Binding — Over the concentration range from 200 to 1,000 ng/mL, approximately 94.5% of fluoxetine is bound in vitro to human serum proteins, including albumin and a1-glycoprotein. The interaction between fluoxetine and other highly protein-bound drugs has not been fully evaluated but may be important (*see* Precautions).

Metabolism — Fluoxetine is extensively metabolized in the liver to norfluoxetine and a number of other, unidentified metabolites. The only identified active metabolite, norfluoxetine, is formed by demethylation of fluoxetine. In animal models, norfluoxetine's potency and selectivity as a serotonin uptake blocker are essentially equivalent to fluoxetine's. The primary route of elimination appears to be hepatic metabolism to inactive metabolites excreted by the kidney.

Clinical Issues Related to Metabolism/Elimination

The complexity of the metabolism of fluoxetine has several consequences that may potentially affect fluoxetine's clinical use.

Accumulation and Slow Elimination — The relatively slow

Clinical Pharmacology of Prozac continued...

elimination of fluoxetine (elimination half-life of two or three days) and its active metabolite, norfluoxetine (elimination half-life of seven to nine days), assures significant accumulation of these active species in chronic use. After 30 days of dosing at 40 mg/day, plasma concentrations of fluoxetine in the range of 91 to 302 ng/mL and norfluoxetine in the range of 72 to 258 ng/mL have been observed. Plasma concentrations of fluoxetine were higher than those predicted by single-dose studies, presumably because fluoxetine's metabolism is not proportional to dose. Norfluoxetine, however, appears to have linear pharmacokinetics. Its mean terminal half-life after a single dose was 8.6 days and after multiple dosing was 9.3 days.

Thus, even if patients are given a fixed dose, steady state plasma concentrations are only achieved after continuous dosing for weeks. Nevertheless, plasma concentrations do not appear to increase without limit. Specifically, patients receiving fluoxetine at dosages of 40 to 80 mg/day over periods as long as three years exhibited, on average, plasma concentrations similar to those seen among patients treated for four or five weeks.

The long elimination half-lives of fluoxetine and norfluoxetine assure that, even when dosing is stopped, active drug substance will persist in the body for weeks. This is of potential consequence when drug discontinuation is required or when drugs are prescribed that might interact with fluoxetine and norfluoxetine following the discontinuation of Prozac.

Liver Disease — As might be predicted from its primary site of metabolism, liver impairment can affect the elimination of fluoxetine. The elimination half-life of fluoxetine was prolonged in a study of cirrhotic patients, with a mean of 7.6 days compared to the range of two to three days seen in subjects without liver disease; norfluoxetine elimination was also delayed, with a mean duration of 12 days for cirrhotic patients compared to the range of seven to nine days in normal subjects. This suggests that the use of fluoxetine in patients with liver disease must be approached with caution. If fluoxetine is administered to patients with liver disease, a lower or less frequent dose should be used (*see* Precautions *and* Dosage and Administration).

Renal Disease — In single-dose studies, the pharmacokinetics of fluoxetine and norfluoxetine were similar among subjects with all levels of impaired renal function, including anephric patients on chronic hemodialysis. However, with chronic administration, additional accumulation of fluoxetine or its metabolites (possibly including some

Clinical Pharmacology of Prozac continued...

not yet identified) may occur in patients with severely impaired renal function, and use of a lower or less frequent dose is advised (*see* Precautions).

Age — The effects of age upon the metabolism of fluoxetine have not been fully explored. The disposition of single doses of fluoxetine in healthy elderly subjects (greater than 65 years of age) did not differ significantly from that in younger normal subjects. However, given the long half-life and nonlinear disposition of the drug, a single-dose study is not adequate to rule out the possibility of altered pharmacokinetics in the elderly, particularly if they have systemic illness or are receiving multiple drugs for concomitant diseases.

Figure 3.4
Role of Tryptophan and other Agents in Depression

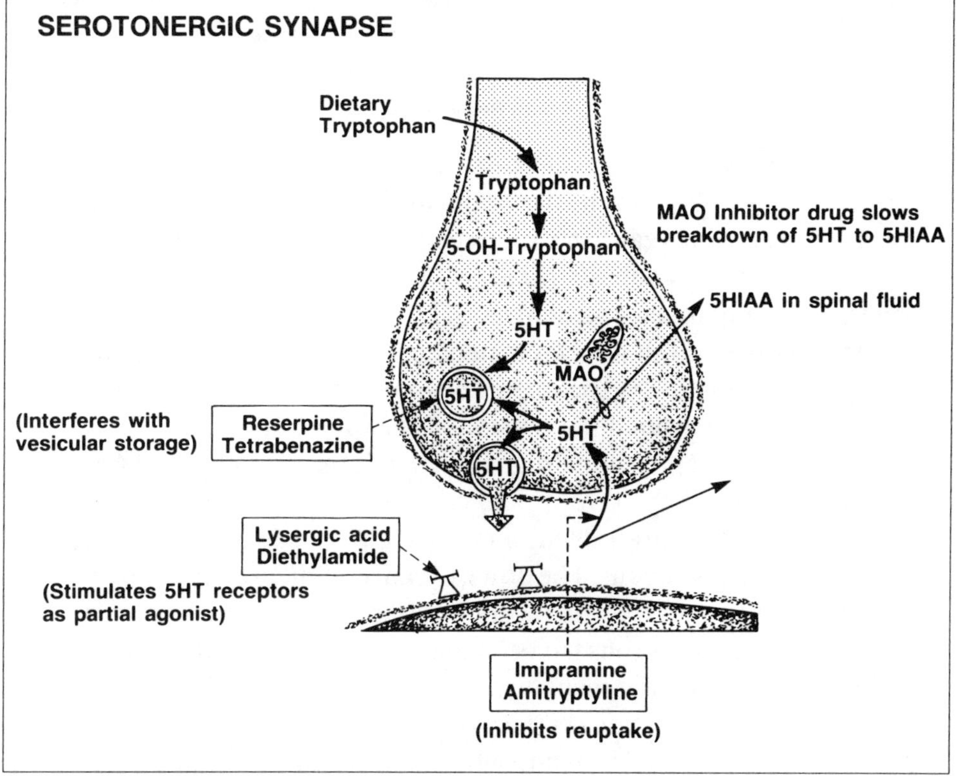

Figure 3.5
Distribution of Serotonin Neurons

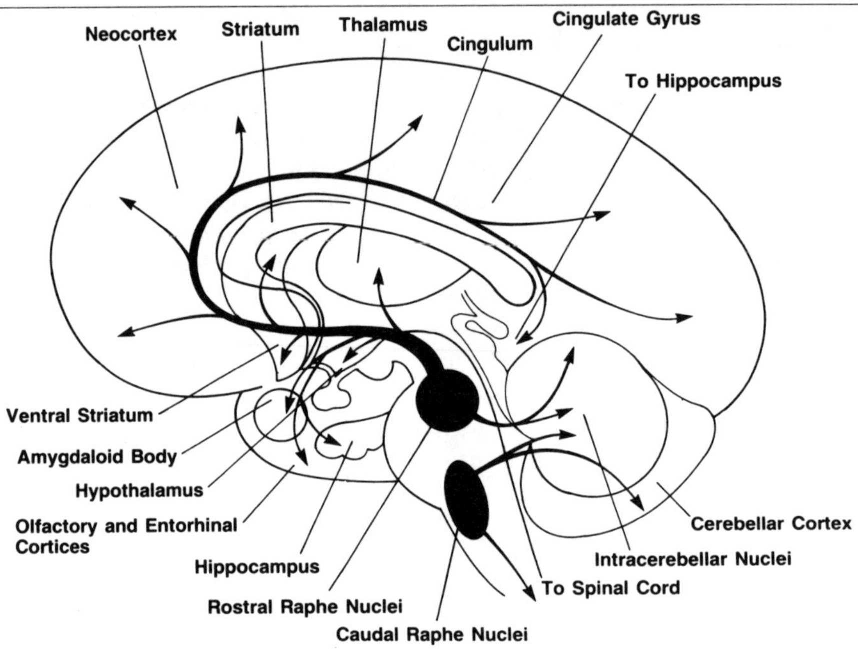

Figure 3.5 puts this discussion is a considerably broader context. It is a diagram of the brain sliced in half, front (left) to back (right), to reveal the structures inside. The dark lines and arrows show the wide distribution of serotonin neurons which release the chemical messenger 5HT (5-hydroxy-tryptophan). Most of these neurons arise from nuclei deep in the brain called the Rostral Raphe Nuclei. The names of some important brain structures are placed around the outside of the diagram for reference.

With antidepression drugs in general, there is a lag of 14 to 21 days before they have a noticeable effect. Pharmacologists think in terms of neurotransmitters having a cascade of effects that take a long time to occur. The downstream chemical changes may actually be the ones that are most important. Another view of this time delay is that neurons have to be sensitized, perhaps they have to be stimulated many, many times before they become activated and continue to function on their own.

Actually, this is similar to what happens during what we call "learning." In the psychologically-oriented therapies, one needs to be sensitized to positive thoughts and desensitized to negative ones. It is well-known that learning in the nervous system occurs by way of multiple electrical stimuli, which eventually produce permanent chemical changes and strengthen connections between certain neurons.

*** Psychological Approaches to Depression

This type of treatment for depression involves being supportive during a crisis or helping the person come to terms with an illness. Those with conflicts and emotional stress related to losses, relationship problems, and poor self-esteem can be helped to understand their inner psychological world and the reasons they are susceptible to depression. Therapy can be guided by several well known approaches to how one should guide others in solving psychological problems:

- **Cognitive therapy** is aimed at breaking a negative pattern of thinking — not transforming it into a Pollyanna outlook, but into a more positive, logical and probably more realistic view of life. A related step is to encourage patients to formulate various ways of looking at their emotional problems, and to examine the implications of each one. The general idea is to promote a sense of competence, leading to greater confidence and a more positive outlook.

- **Behavioral therapy** often involves getting patients to take part in activities which clearly help break away from behaviors which need changing. The focus here is usually quite specific, and there is often little concern about the deeper emotional traumas which may have generated a behavior. The goal is to define a specific problem and attack it scientifically and directly via techniques such as:

- *systematic desensitization*, generally involving a step-by-step substitution of relaxation for anxiety
- *modeling*, or learning to change via the direct observation of others
- *behavior rehearsal* generally involving role-playing
- *positive reinforcement*
- *self-regulation* via the careful monitoring of one's own behavior

- **Family or couples therapy** is helpful to those needing to deal with difficulties in their relationships;

- **Group therapy** helps people in the same boat productively share their experiences or fears usually involving a similar problem.

Sometimes a combination of several of these techniques works best.

There is considerable debate in psychiatry as to whether drug therapy or cognitive-psychological is best, and in some cases it would appear that both are effective. However, there is a certain type of depression in which drugs or ECT are necessary. This is when the problem involves a change in mood, and a slowing down of motor and vegetative functions, quite independent of any change in thinking or self-esteem.

*** *Electroconvulsive Therapy (ECT)*

As mentioned earlier in chapter one, ECT has of course aroused much controversy and criticism. Nonetheless it indeed can be effective when various psychological approaches or anti-depressant medications are not having the desired effect, or when there is some physical condition, such as heart disease, that can make various psychotropic drugs hazardous. For those whose depression is so severe their lives may be at stake, ECT also can bring fast results, long before drugs can be effective. Its side effects include

Figure 3.6
Modern Machine Used in Electroconvulsive Therapy
As Illustrated in a Technical Ad Directed at Psychiatrists

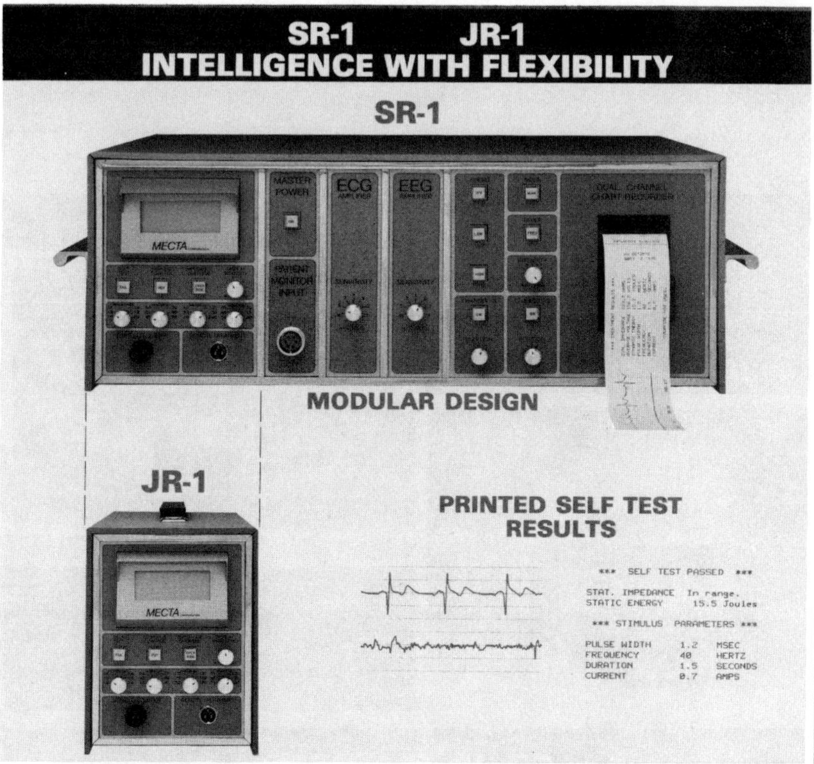

transient headaches, and temporary short-term memory loss.

With the modern equipment available today there are no absolute situations in which ECT should not be used, but there are cases in which there is an increased risk. Patients with brain tumors and those with stroke may suffer further brain damage from ECT, but there are measures to counteract these effects, which are usually transient. The patient with a recent heart attack or severe high blood pressure may be at risk because ECT markedly raises blood pressure temporarily. The field of ECT has quite a bit more history than most people suspect, and it has certainly evolved dramatically from its early applications. The picture in figure 3.8 illustrate the now primitive-appearing conditions under which it was first practiced, in 1938, in Italy.

Figure 3.7
Ad Detailing the Features of a Modern ETC Machine

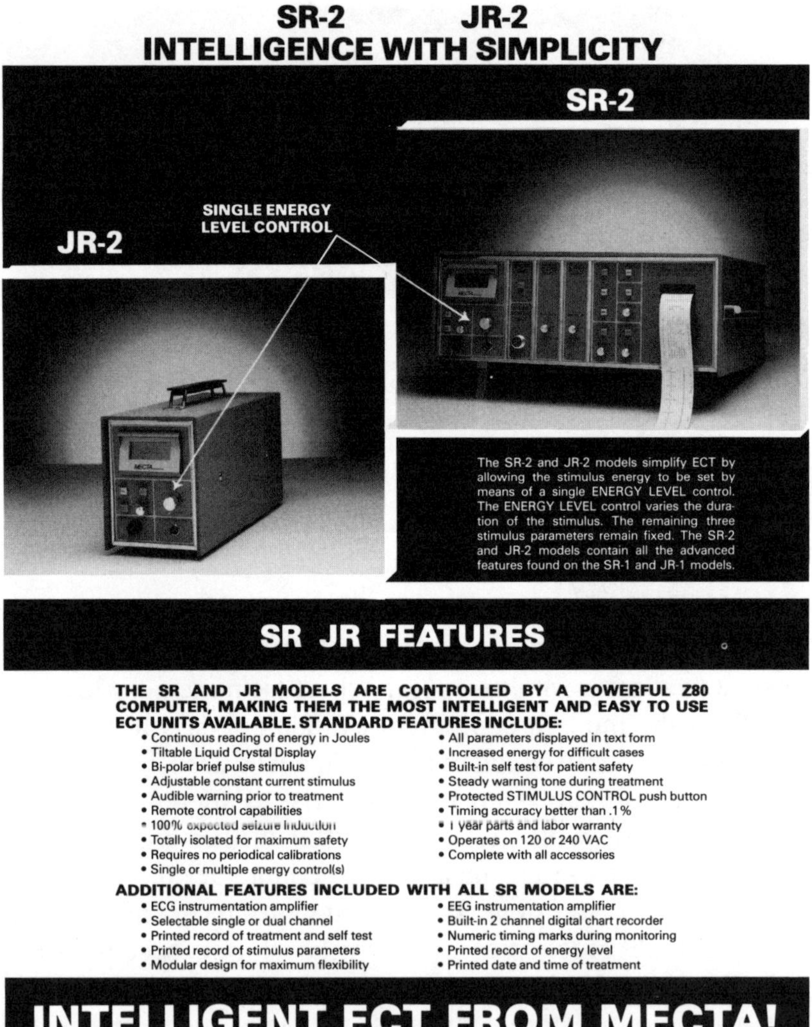

Figure 3.8
Photographs of Setting Where ECT was First Employed

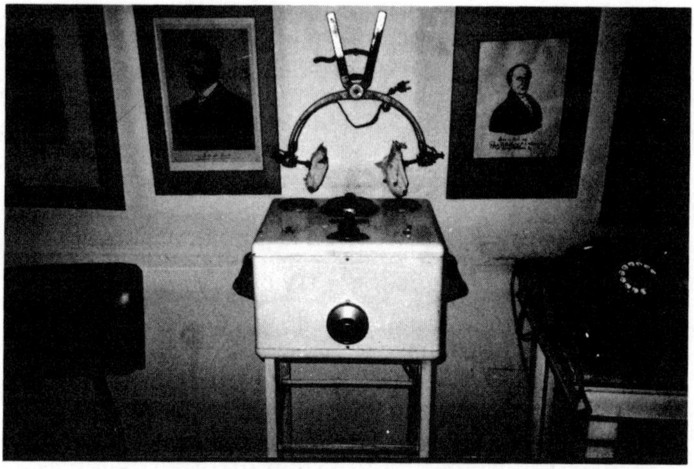

The original electroshock therapy apparatus used in 1938, now in the History of Medicine Museum in Rome (Photograph by Norman S. Endler, October 1985)

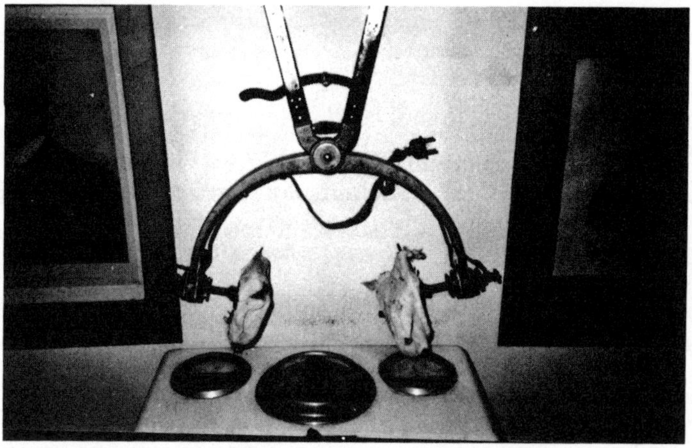

Electrodes used in the first electroshock treatment in 1938, now in the History of Medine Museum in Rome (Photograph by Norman S. Endler, October 1985)

Source: Endler, N. (1988). *Electroconvulsive Therapy: The Myths and the Realities.* Toronto: Hogrefe & Huber Publishers.

Broader Social Solutions to Depression

In addition, social and community approaches can include instruction in improving coping skills, help in developing supportive relationships, involvement of community agencies, and education about affective disorders. Doctors and therapists often refer patients who have recovered from depression to a variety of social agencies for counseling on couple or family problems, as well as training on how to be more assertive and self-respecting. In addition, courses on effective parenting are available in many communities through public and private sector agencies or community colleges.

Overall, early diagnosis and effective treatment can be crucial in preventing the depressed person from acting on his suicidal thoughts, or dying from physical deterioration.

It is also important that physical disorders such as anemia and thyroid disease, which may cause some of the same symptoms, be ruled out early in the treatment of the person exhibiting characteristics of depression.

*** Research

One of the major needs in this field today is to develop better ways of predicting which persons will actually benefit from the various medications now available; which persons will respond best to psychotherapies; and in which cases a combination of treatments would be best.

Most people can discontinue their anti-depressant medications after three to six months and do not relapse. However, some people do, and therefore require long-term treatment with these drugs, which then involves dealing with their various side effects. This is why much more information is needed on the safety and optimal duration of long-term treatment. More knowledge of how brain chemistry controls mood could lead to anti-depressants that act in hours or days, rather than weeks or months.

For example, one study has shown that simply depriving a person of the substance tryptophan in the diet gradually leads to mild depression. Tryptophan is merely a normal dietary amino acid needed for the chemical synthesis of serotonin in the brain. In this connection there is now a major ongoing search to find a way to boost serotonin's action more quickly than current anti-depressants do. Fluoxetine (Prozac), described above, acts like serotonin, but its action is delayed.

It also would be a major advance if ways could be found to protect people who have risk factors for affective disorders from becoming ill in the first place. Elderly people who are beset by loneliness and a sense of meaninglessness, and single mothers with several children and no one to confide in or lean on, are both very commonly at risk for depression. Formal social experiments in which people in these two sets of circumstances were brought together to artificially reproduce an extended family might be worthwhile as a treatment of several problems at once.

Recent research on factors that influence changes in mood, such as light and temperature, promises to clarify the reasons for shifts in the mood. A new type of light bulb has been developed, for example, that appears to reduce the effects of Seasonal Affective Disorder.

Some chromosome-containing genes that cause depression in some people have recently been discovered. We need to identify these genes and know how they produce the abnormal chemicals in the brain that ultimately lower mood to devastating depths.

*** *For Further Information*

Associations

Depression/Awareness, Recognition, Treatment (D/ART), National Institute of Mental Health, Rockville, MD 20857
National Depressive and Manic Depressive Association, 53 West Jackson Blvd. Box USN, Chicago, Illinois 60604.

National Mental Health Association Information Center, 1021 Prince Street, Alexandria, VA 22314.

The National Foundation for Depressive Illness, PO Box 2257 New York, New York.

The National Association for Research on Schizophrenia and Depression, 60 Cutter Mill Road, Suite 200, Great Neck, New York 11021.

Books

Burns, D. (1981). *Feeling Good.* New York: Signet.

Emery, G. (1988). *Getting Undepressed.* Toronto: Simon and Schuster Ltd.

Fieve, R.R. (1975). *Mood Swing.* New York: Bantam Books. (Focuses on manic-depressive illness).

Gillett, R. (1987). Overcoming *Depression: A Practical Self Help Guide to Prevention and Treatment.* Toronto: MacMillan Canada Ltd.

Klein, D.F. and Wender, P.H. (1988). *Do You Have Depressive Illness? How to Tell, What to Do.* New York: Plume.

Chapter 4

Anxiety Disorders

Suppose that while walking down the street, you are suddenly confronted by a big, snarling dog. Your heart starts to pound, your muscles tighten, your mouth goes dry, your breathing speeds up. You are experiencing a natural fear reaction geared to prepare the body for fight or flight: to get away from the situation as quickly as possible, or stand your ground and battle it out.

While all of us experience fear or anxiety or have simple phobias, such as the fear of snakes, as part of our normal survival mechanisms, they are abnormal only when they are persistent and disruptive and there is no appropriate reason for them.

Statistics show that at about 8.3 percent of the people in North America at some time in their lives suffer from conditions called anxiety disorders. This may seem to be a relatively modest figure, but it represents some 23 million people.

Some sufferers have a "generalized anxiety disorder," where for months they have been nervous, anxious or worried about some possible, but undefined, misfortune to themselves or others. When anxious, they may feel shaky, dizzy, nauseous, on edge, restless and irritable. Palpitations, sore muscles, shortness of breath, sweaty or clammy hands, diarrhea, and hot flashes or chills can be among their symptoms.

"Agoraphobia" describes the condition where people's lives are increasingly restricted as they become unwilling to simply go outside of their houses, due to a fear of open spaces. This term is derived from the Greek words for marketplace and fear. This particular version of panic disorder is often the most difficult, because it can result in people being completely housebound.

But it is now recognized that it is not the "marketplace" or any other public place itself which they fear, but the possibility that they may suffer a panic attack in a situation where it is hard to escape, or help might not be available. They can still have these attacks at home, and even be awakened from sleep by them.

Unpredictably, and in completely normal circumstances, the victims of this disorder are suddenly overwhelmed by panic: heart palpitations, sweating, dizziness, trembling, faintness. They stand gasping, terrified of losing control, afraid that they are going crazy, or going to die. These attacks usually last only a few minutes, but in rare cases can go on for hours.

The half-filled grocery cart found abandoned in an aisle at closing time was more likely left by a woman trying to flee a panic attack than one who suddenly discovered her wallet was at home.

Arnold was a 30-year-old accountant who went to his doctor complaining of extreme fear, sweating, shortness of breath, palpitations, chest pain and headaches. Blood tests, a physical examination and electrocardiograph turned up nothing. He and his wife, also an accountant, had been happily married for three years and had an active social life, but because of his attacks he started to avoid driving, and asked her to accompany him everywhere. Eventually, he couldn't bring himself to go to work, and took a medical leave of absence.

He told his doctor the attacks had started about the time he and his wife had started talking about buying a house and having children, and eventually he admitted he was intimidated by these responsibilities. He responded to three weeks' treatment with "Imipramine," combined with psychotherapy to help him find ways of dealing with his fear of greater responsibility.

In addition he was given a course of behavioral and cognitive therapy to desensitize him to his fear of leaving home. After a few months he recovered, and returned to a more normal life, having become convinced that he could handle his impending new responsibilities.

Over the years, lists of dozens of phobias have been compiled: claustrophobia, or fear of enclosed spaces, is well known, and children have fun pronouncing "triskaidekaphobia," or fear of the number 13. Some are obscure indeed: "siderodromophobia" for fear of railways, "osmophobia" for fear of odors, and "belonophobia" for fear of pins.

Psychiatrists now lump these together under "simple phobias" — persistent unreasonable fear of a specific object or situation. It may be a fear of heights, the dark, a certain animal, bird or insect, the sight of blood or driving across any bridge.

A young married professional woman developed a fear of grasshoppers in her early teens, and by the time she was in her 20s, she was unable to enjoy the outdoors in summer. She was always on the lookout for grasshoppers, drove with her windows tightly closed, and tried to avoid the occasional field trips her job required. This phobia, of course, eventually affected her social life, her job, and her self-esteem.

There are also social phobias, where the person fears he — and it's more often he — will be embarrassed or humiliated. This is much more than the transient "butterflies" most people feel before making a speech or appearing on stage. It is an intense anxiety that causes marked distress, and can be brought on by eating in restaurants or going to a social gathering. Because the person avoids or just tries to endure these situations, it can interfere with his social life and/or his career.

"Post-traumatic stress disorder" follows a traumatic event, but the panic attacks involved often occur in situations completely unrelated to the original trauma.

An example of such a disorder is the sales clerk who was

twice assaulted during robberies at a variety store. She has not been able to return to her job a year after the second attack, even though she has recovered from the physical aspects of the ordeal. She avoids going out at night, complains of neck pains, is relying on Valium, and has panic attacks even in the safety of her own home. Her sleep is persistently troubled by nightmares in which she sees the hooded head of a robber coming towards her, and wakes up panicky and terrified.

This disorder became more widely recognized after experience with Vietnam veterans in the United States, and an increasing number of cases are being described by victims of rapes and assaults.

Another problem of this general type is "obsessive compulsive disorder" wherein people devise repetitive, complicated rituals, and fear some catastrophe if they do not follow them exactly. They may repeatedly check things, like going the rounds of all the door and window locks three times before going to bed. They may be obsessed with "germs," and repeatedly wash and disinfect things, like the telephone receiver, after every use. They may find it impossible to take a detour if there's been an accident on their usual route to work.

Many of the costs to society of these disorders are hidden. The person may go from doctor to doctor, fearing that the physical symptoms of a panic attacks are due to some serious disease like a heart condition or multiple sclerosis, and demanding more and more tests to find it. On the other hand, if phobias involve illness, needles or blood, the person may avoid getting medical or dental attention in the early stages of disease.

It has recently been found that one-third of alcohol abusers have anxiety disorders, raising the possibility that treatment for anxiety could prevent some alcoholism, or improve the outcome for some alcoholics.

Although women are considered to be more susceptible to all these disorders except social phobias, it may be that the true incidence in men is masked by alcohol abuse. As one doctor put it in describing coping patterns, "Men are more likely to go to the liquor store than the doctor."

Broken marriages and lost jobs are part of the toll. Since the most severe anxiety disorders tend to occur in young adults, when they are making important life decisions, many never reach their potential for a fulfilling career and family life. As in the case of schizophrenia, this situation makes the overall cost to society much higher than if these problems occurred only in much older people.

*** Causes

Fingers point in many directions when the causes of anxiety disorders are being sought — as in many other mental conditions, there is probably a mixture of factors that varies from one person to another.

Genetics may play a role for some: studies have shown that on average, 17 percent of close relatives of people with panic disorder are also diagnosed with it.

At present very little is known about how anxiety and phobias could be transmitted by parents, or engendered by childhood experiences. Children may adopt fearful behavior which they see in their parents, but there is no proof that this causes disorders when they are adults. Most childhood fears which are within the range of normal, like fear of the dark, go away spontaneously.

However, there does seem to be an association between adolescent school phobias and adult anxiety disorders. Many affected adults recall episodes of separation and humiliation during their development. Others had stressful events months before the onset of symptoms.

There are also biological possibilities. With the new brain imaging techniques, such as positron emission tomography (PET) scans, researchers can see the functioning of the brain, not just its static physical structure.

Some scientists are using these and other techniques to solve this problem by studying the small "locus ceruleus" at the base of the brain — it gets its name from the Latin for blue because it has a bluish tinge. As illustrated in Figure 4.1, it gives rise to nerve fibers that travel to almost every region of the cortex, the outer

Figure 4.1
Locus Ceruleus and Associated Aspects of the Brain

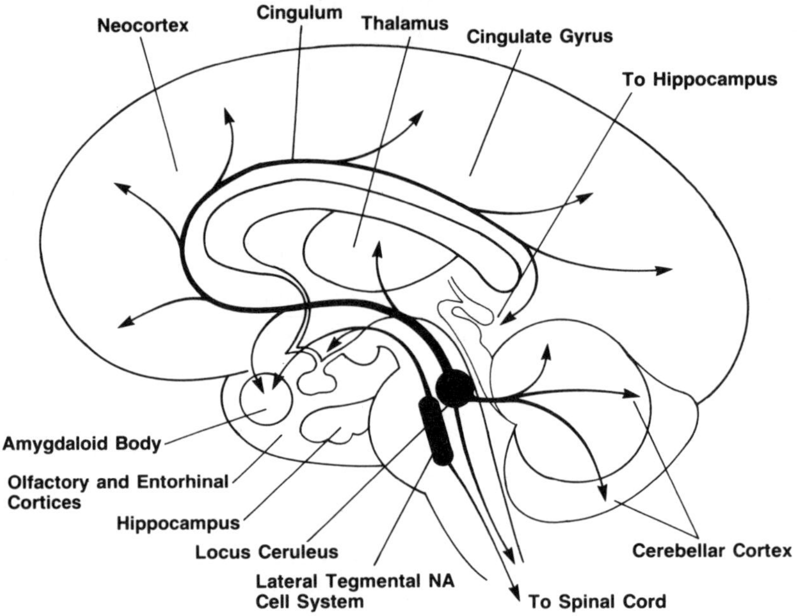

layers of the two hemispheres of the brain.

Over-stimulation of that nucleus will cause increased activity throughout the brain, and a sense of panic or total fear. Lesser anxiety, such as that involved in anticipation of a possible threat, may involve only a subset of those fibers, and has been shown to increase activity in the temporal lobes. Drugs that suppress this area reduce anxiety, and those that stimulate it can produce an anxiety that is almost panic.

There was once a fad of attributing anxiety symptoms to hypoglycemia, or low blood sugar. In an insulin-dependent diabetic whose blood sugar drops when he hasn't eaten, the dizziness, trembling, disorientation and rapid heart rate of an insulin reaction are symptoms similar to a panic attack. This is an interesting observation, but, when blood sugar is measured during anxiety attacks per se, it turns out to be normal.

Hormonal changes have been suggested as a factor in the onset of anxiety disorders in women, since many of them get their first panic attack after changes involving hormonal fluctuations, such as childbirth, miscarriage, menopause, and pre-menstrual periods. Nonetheless, so far no clearly viable results have emerged from these studies.

Hyperventilation or over-breathing accompanies some panic attacks. Recent research has indicated that some people with anxiety are chronic hyperventilators, although this isn't obvious to a casual observer. These victims can produce the chemical changes of hyperventilation by breathing a little more deeply or rapidly. The research has also indicated that many of these people can be helped simply by learning controlled breathing techniques.

In some people, panic attacks can be precipitated by the use of illicit drugs such as cocaine, marijuana or amphetamines, or by the caffeine in coffee, tea or cola drinks, and those with anxiety disorders should certainly avoid all of these relatively high-risk substances.

*** Treatment

Anxiety disorders have one of the brighter treatment pictures in psychiatry. Up to two-thirds of people with them may improve without treatment of any kind, although this may take several years, whereas specific therapy can often work much faster. In general a combination of medication and psychotherapy is used.

In particular, some helpful treatments include:

- programs that gradually expose the person to mild forms of the things or situations he fears
- imaging exercises where the victim thinks of appropriate responses when confronted with what he fears
- detailed relaxation techniques, and
- systematic training to avoid catastrophic thinking.

These desensitization and relaxation techniques were introduced by psychologists and are utilized by many of them in helping their patients. Increasingly, psychiatrists have been learning the value of these methods and there are now many anxiety disorder clinics where psychiatrists, psychologists, nurses and social workers teach such techniques to patients, with quite good effects. Involvement of the family, and participation in support groups can also be very helpful.

Drugs such as tranquillizers and anti-depressants may be a necessary part of anti-anxiety therapy. However, just why they work in some anxiety states is not yet clear. Tranquillizers such as Valium are also effective. Valium has a particularly long period of action — it takes about 48 hours for 50% of it to be eliminated from the body — so it may be preferable to shorter-acting drugs like lorazepam, which is sold under the trade name Ativan.

The following brief excerpt is from the *Clinical Handbook of Psychropic Drugs*, which we have discussed earlier. The extract in this case shows the first of many tables which deal with the significant characteristics and interactions of the major anxiolytic drugs. While many of these medications are well-known and often appear to be similar, their effects differ widely, as can be seen here.

Unfortunately, there is a risk of physical and/or psychological dependence, or even addiction with these drugs. In particular, some degree of dependence is possible if they are taken daily for more than three weeks. In the past, and to a lesser extent now, they have been over-prescribed.

A study at Dartmouth Medical School, recently discussed in the relatively new magazine *Longevity*, points out a further hazard of tranquilizer use over a long period of time. The subjects studied over a 40-year span, all male, had used tranquillizers, sleeping pills and anti-depressants regularly from their 20s through their 50s, and were found to develop ill health and psychological problems as they entered their 60s. Remarkably, tranquillizer use was found to be more significant than smoking, overweight, stress and drinking as a potential cause of poor physical and mental health at age 65. The root cause here may be the problems that led to the use of tranquillizers in the first place. The psychiatrist, George Vaillant, has followed a large number of people for decades in this regard. Those who had psychological problems, not illnesses, that they never solved in life tended to get medical

Table 4.1
Comparison of Major Anti-Anxiety Medications

Drug	Equivalent Dose (mg)**	Peak Plasma Level p.o.	Elimination Half-life	Metabolites (m = main metabolite)	Comments	Clinically Significant Interactions	Clinical Considerations
Alprazolam	0.5	1 - 2 hrs	9 - 20 hrs	29 metabolites; principal ones are: α-hydroxyalprazolam desmethylalprazolam 4-hydroxyalprazolam	Rapidly and completely absorbed 80% protein bound α-hydroxyalprazolam is active	Probably similar to diazepam	Use: anxiolytic sedative alcohol withdrawal depression characterized by anxiety Panic attack prophylaxis t.i.d. dosing recommended Increases stage 2, and decreases stages 1 & 4 and REM sleep Caution on withdrawal
Bromazepam	3.0	0.5 - 4 hrs	12 hrs mean	3-hydroxybromazepam (8 - 19 hrs)	Metabolite reported to have anxiolytic activity	CNS depressants: increased effect on the CNS *	Use: anxiolytic Not recommended for use in patients with depressive disorders or psychoses *
Chlordiaz-epoxide	25.0	1 - 4 hrs	14 hrs mean (4 - 29 hrs parent drug) (28 - 100 hrs metabolites)	desmethylchlor-diazepoxide (m) demoxepam desoxydemoxepam	Volume of distribution (Vd) significantly larger in young females than males Elimination half-life prolonged and total plasma clearance decreased in elderly men (less so in elderly women)	Antacids:* decrease absorption in GI tract, but do not influence completeness of absorption Cimetidine:* increases blood levels of chlordiazepoxide by decreasing elimination	Use: anxiolytic sedative alcoholism treatment 2 to 3-fold increase in half-life seen in patients with cirrhosis
Clonazepam	0.25	1 - 4 hrs	34 hrs mean (19 - 60 hrs)	No active metabolite	Quickly and completely absorbed		Use: anticonvulsant, mostly in childhood seizures such as myoclonic infantile spasms and absences Panic attack prophylaxis Manic episode of B.A.D.
Clorazepate dipotassium	10.0	variable	1.3 - 96 hrs metabolites	N-desmethyldiazepam (m)	Hydrolyzed in the stomach to active metabolite (parent compound inactive) Rate of hydrolysis depends on gastric acidity, therefore absorption is unreliable (one study disputes this)	Antacids & Sodium Bicarbonate: reduce the rate and extent of appearance of active metabolite in the blood	Use: anxiolytic

Source: Bezchlibnyk-Butler, K. and Jeffries, J. (1990) *Clinical Handbook of Psychotropic Drugs.* Hogrefe & Huber Publishers: Toronto.

illnesses in their 60's — more often than less unhappy people.

While the dependence involved with these medications is not as severe as with narcotics, it is a good idea for patients to take drug holidays, such as three weeks on, and then a week off. If a drug must be continued for longer periods, it should be discontinued very gradually over a period of days or weeks to prevent withdrawal effects. These effects are usually mild, unless high doses have been taken, but they involve insomnia and so-called rebound anxiety.

Anti-anxiety drugs of course should not be dispensed as though they were candy, even though they are among the safest medications we have, and there may be a temptation for some busy doctors to hand them out too readily. On the other hand, many physicians may have become too cautious about using them, leaving patients to continue suffering needlessly.

* * * Research

The science of psychotherapy itself certainly needs further refinement, since about one-third of patients who undergo this treatment do not obtain optimal results. In addition there is still a need for drugs which do not have a potential for dependence.

In the past few years several techniques, such as breathing carbon dioxide or injecting lactate, have been developed to produce panic attacks in the laboratory, so they can be studied more easily. Voluntary hyperventilation can also produce panic attacks in some susceptible people.

New inventions have enabled scientists to better monitor heart and breathing functions while people go about their normal activities. These have added to our knowledge of anxiety symptoms outside the laboratory.

Behavior therapy for phobic avoidance has been improved through many research studies in the past decade. Most of them have concentrated on refining exposure techniques:

- how long and how frequently the person should be exposed to what is feared

- whether drugs should also be used
- whether it is helpful to have a companion or a therapist present during exposure

Relaxation techniques for treatment of general anxiety have also been well-researched. Very recently, the cognitive and the controlled breathing treatment of panic has also received a great deal of research attention, with promising results.

A key to better medications may lie in research on the biology involved in the suppression of anxiety: the "benzodiazepine receptor system." It is known that these drugs work when attracted to receptors on the surfaces of some nerve cells, but not how or why. What is the original purpose of the receptors? Obviously, Mother Nature did not put them there to sit idle until man invented Valium. Understanding the basic mechanisms of this system and its interactions with others could open many more therapeutic doors.

Obsessive-compulsive disorders apparently involve a different chemical receptor in the brain, called 5-HT, even though they are also associated with anxiety and fear. An alternative type of drug, fluoxetine (Prozac) described in the chapter on depression, that affects this particular type of receptor seems to work best for this disorder, and the nature of this mechanism needs to be much more fully understood.

Remarkably, despite the number of people with these problems, and the amount of money spent on various medications, the relative efficacy of tranquillizers, anti-depressants and cognitive therapy have not yet been thoroughly compared. Of course, this major piece of research would be most valuable, especially considering the increasing financial pressures on both government and private health care systems.

*** For Further Information

The Freedom From Fear Foundations, founded in Toronto in 1974 as a self-help group, now has chapters in many cities.

Greist, J.W. and Jefferson, J.W. and Marks, I.M. (1986). *Anxiety and its Treatment: Help is Available*, Washington: American Psychiatric Press.

Marks, I.M. (1978). *Living with Fear, Understanding and Coping with Anxiety*, New York: MacGraw-Hill.

Weeks, Claire.(1978). *Hope and Help for your Nerves*, New York: Bantam Books.

Chapter 5

Personality Disorders

Psychiatrists sometimes envy the diagnostic tools of their medical colleagues: an X-ray that determines if a bone is fractured, a urine test that announces pregnancy, a blood test that points to diabetes, a CAT scan that shows a tumor.

Mental illnesses are not always clear-cut, and nowhere is that more obvious than in the group of conditions called personality disorders.

All of us have peculiar personality traits that irritate or frustrate our friends, relatives and colleagues. All of us see habits in ourselves that we don't like. However, when these traits seriously interfere with our functioning and development, when they consistently make people around us miserable, they get labelled as personality disorders.

It's a difficult diagnostic process: like judging where on a scale of one to 10 is it best to stop saying "that's normal" and start saying "that's sick." You can't be a little bit pregnant, but personality disorders are a matter of degree. Yet with training, different psychiatrists who see the same person often have a high degree of agreement in their diagnosis regarding this problem.

In general, individuals with these conditions have inflexible and unproductive patterns of behavior and ways of thinking that are consistent over time — they tend to behave in a way that is self-detrimental, in spite of the consequences that behavior has brought in the past.

Their relationships with others tend to be shallow or chaotic, and their educational and work achievement levels are often lower than would be expected from their intelligence levels. They may be more prone to develop other psychiatric illnesses because of the stress imposed by their relationships with others, and the inappropriate ways they perceive and cope with adverse events in their lives.

Efforts to bring some scientific order to the diagnosis and treatment of these problems have resulted in a list of disorders that assembles patterns of behavior and symptoms under different categories. Not all psychiatrists agree on what constitutes a specific disorder, and human personalities, in their infinite variety, don't fit neatly into diagnostic cubicles. To add to the complexity, people with many other psychiatric problems may also have a personality disorder.

In any case, these many variations of the problem have been grouped together in clusters, each containing several different labels, but each of them sharing some features.

One of these categories is the "odd cluster," which includes paranoid and schizotype personality disorders. These people have a very restricted range of emotional expression, and a high level of mistrust and aloofness when dealing with others. Almost everyone knows someone who has these personality traits. But having a trait is different from having a personality disorder, though there are not yet any scientific criteria distinguishing one from the other.

A second category is the "dramatic cluster," those who overdramatize, exaggerate, and go to extremes to attract attention. They include borderline, antisocial, histrionic and narcissistic personality disorders.

The third group are the "anxious cluster," and include avoidant, dependent, impulsive and passive aggressive personality disorders. These people are often anxious, and behave in ways to attempt to reduce that anxiety:

- avoiding social situations in the avoidant personality disorder
- avoiding decision-making for fear of making mistakes in the compulsive personality disorder
- remaining subordinate to others in the dependent

personality disorder
- procrastinating rather than expressing resentment in the passive aggressive personality disorder.

There are gender differences in expression of various disorders, but they lie in gender differences per se, and are not inherent in the disorder. For example, antisocial behavior in men is most apt to involve aggression and alcohol, while women are more likely to use their sexuality. Antisocial personality disorders may be four times more frequent in men than women, whereas histrionic disorder is more commonly found in women.

Major studies in the past have identified personality disorders in 6 to 10% of the population, but they did not distinguish clearly between traits and disorders, and they did not specify which types were more prevalent.

Here is a sampling of symptoms of a few of the labelled personality disorders: it is important to keep in mind that it is the combination of traits, the severity and consistency of them that denote illness.

Avoidant Personality Disorder

These people are so constantly worried and insecure that they avoid any situation or relationship that they think will underline their inadequacies. They tend to stay on the fringe, alert for signs of rejection or ridicule. They want affection and acceptance, but are afraid to get involved with other people unless they have almost a written guarantee of uncritical acceptance. Their self-esteem is so low they make a big deal of their shortcomings and can't give themselves credit for a job well done.

A 25-year-old electrician was referred to a psychologist because of an upsurge in anxiety after another man with less seniority had been promoted over him. He thought this might be due, in part, to the fact that he avoided involvement with other people, even though he very much wanted to be part of the in-group at the plant. He hesitated to join in unless invited, feeling he didn't have much to offer and would probably be rejected anyway. He had always been shy as a youth, and although he had two good friends, he was known as a loner.

A number of interesting recent studies have shown that shy children show more physical reactions, such as heart rate and perspiration, to new situations than other children. This is not a mental illness, but a variation in personal responsiveness. Nonetheless, without special encouragement and gradual introduction to novel situations, such children can possibly become avoidant personalities.

For the electrician, treatment in therapy sessions involved rehearsals of scenes where he joined in with other people, and in this relaxed atmosphere he gradually became less sensitive and more sociable.

Antisocial Personality Disorder

People with this more severe problem are at war with the world. Even at a very early age, they were disasters at school — a litany of truancy, expulsions, suspensions, lying, starting fights, ignoring all the rules, and getting grades far below their potential followed them through their school days. Outside school, life wasn't much better: patterns of delinquency, alcohol or other drug abuse, vandalism, or running away from home have been revealed.

As these people become adults, the problem does not change, but only takes on more adult forms: high absenteeism from work, job-hopping, long spells of unemployment. Rules and responsibilities mean nothing. Children can be abused or neglected, people conned, money squandered, spouses deserted.

Arnie, who was being interviewed by a psychiatrist while in jail awaiting trial for robbery, was typical. At 20, he already had a long history of trouble, like car theft and other robberies. He had been expelled from school for fighting and destroying property, and when he was out in a vocational training program, he ran away in two weeks. Juvenile courts sent him to various institutions, from which he also ran away. He was not close to his brother or sister, or any friends.

Unlike people with avoidant personality, boys like Arnie are highly insensitive to social events, particularly punishment. They do not learn from experience. Scientists are working on the theory that there are reward and punishment systems in the brain, and the chemical systems involved may be badly deranged in these people, but the details of such a defect are not yet known.

Borderline Personality Disorders

People with this problem are over-reactors, who can fly into a rage at a perceived slight or criticism. When they are emotionally upset, they feel like they are falling apart, and they are not able to think logically about solutions to problems. They often feel empty and bored and "not together," and will seek extreme sensations to make them feel "whole" — or feel anything at all. They can go on sprees of eating, sex, spending, gambling, drugs, or cut their wrists. Many of them turn to drugs for solace, which often results in a further downward spiral of stress, financial pressures and failure.

Paradoxically, they can not stand being alone, yet their behavior makes it impossible for them to sustain lasting relationships with others. They can go from a normal mood to depression, irritability or anxiety that lasts for several hours, then disappears.

Debbie was admitted to a hospital at 26 because of her intense suicidal urges, and her self-mutilation with a razor. She had been well until her mid-teens when she began to avoid her friends and became filled with doubts about who she was. She went to college and did quite well academically, but she began to take a variety of drugs and associated with a charismatic cult figure on the campus. She found her waves of intense anxiety would vanish if she slashed her arm with a razor blade.

At first, she thought her therapist at the college counseling service was the most intuitive human on earth, then she became disappointed in his "lack of understanding" and became increasingly demanding, insisting on two or more sessions a day. When she wasn't in his office, she felt intensely and unbearably alone.

Margo also had this aversion to being alone, and by age 30, she had a long series of boyfriends and one husband. She was forever falling in and out of love, quickly coming to hate the man with whom she had thought herself happy, and being extremely critical of him. If he dropped her, she'd mix Valium and alcohol to try and kill herself, and eventually she began taking Valium daily in ever-increasing doses.

Dependent Personality Disorder

People in this category cling to others for dear life. They cannot function independently, and let someone else assume the responsibility for everything from the dinner menu to what kind of job they should seek. These people think of themselves as helpless and stupid. They will go to any lengths — even tolerate physical abuse — to meet the needs of the people they depend upon, so they won't have to rely on themselves or take responsibility for their own decisions.

Tony, a 34-year-old carpenter, has broken up with his girlfriend because his mother doesn't want him to marry her. He has never lived away from home, and he complains that his mother is hanging on to him and will never let him marry. He is afraid of her for criticizing him, but he also admires and respects her, and generally allows her to wear the pants in the family. He figures she was probably right — his girlfriend wasn't the right mate for him.

As the youngest of three children, he was babied and spoiled by his mother and sisters. He had difficulty getting to sleep if his mother didn't stay in his room; he had problems being left alone at school; and he was unbearably homesick at a sleep-over at another boy's home.

Paranoid Personality Disorder

Pay this person a compliment, and he wonders what your ulterior motive is. Point out a mistake, and he'll find 17 reasons why he's not to blame.

This is not the severe mental disorder of paranoid schizophrenia, where hallucinations and bizarre plots are perceived as threatening. Instead this problem involves those who expect people are going to trick them, who are always on the lookout for hidden motives and special meanings, but pride themselves on always being objective, rational and unemotional. Yet they are quick to take offense and can be "insanely" jealous.

But the disorder can also be more subtle. A social worker in a retirement home was assessing the needs of a 70-year-old man who seemed moderately guarded and didn't reveal anything about himself. His daughter said he had always believed himself to be immune to problems, and he thought he acted only on the basis of rational thought. His wife was probably the only person he ever trusted, and he had carefully cared for her. He never revealed himself to others, assuming they were out to get something from him, and if a friend sincerely offered help, he would suspiciously refuse it. He hid receipts and "evidence" in his safety deposit box to prepare for the eventuality of law suits over trivial matters.

Schizoid Personality Disorder

The schizoid personality seems flat, even icy. Distant and aloof, he feels no warmth or tenderness toward others, and has no sensitivity to their feelings. He couldn't care less if others praise or criticize him.

> *Leonard, a 30-year-old lawyer, was dragged to a marriage counselor by his wife because he wouldn't join in family activities, showed little interest in the children and displayed no affection. His job involved looking up information in law libraries, so he had little contact with his colleagues—they considered him shy or aloof. He told the therapist he only got married to please his parents. Despite his detachment, there was no indication that he was depressed.*

The schizotypal can also be cold and aloof, with few if any close friends. But he can be hypersensitive to real or imagined criticism, and suspicious of others.

He may be superstitious, think he is clairvoyant or telepathic, and feel the presence of people not actually there. His speech may be odd — not incoherent, but vague, over-elaborate, and often distinctly wandering.

Narcissistic Personality Disorder

This one gets its name from the beautiful youth Narcissus in Greek mythology, who fell in love with his image in a pool, and pined away because they couldn't get together. People with this disorder have an exaggerated sense of their own importance or uniqueness, and can spend hours fantasizing about their success, beauty and power. They need constant attention and admiration, and expect everyone to do favors for them, without ever expecting anything in return. They can be users who take advantage of others to get what they want, and are unable to understand how other people feel. If criticized, bested or ignored by others, they can react with cool indifference, or feel enraged and humiliated.

James is a 27-year-old neurosciences student who believes he has developed an understanding of brain function that makes him unique, and that he has a theory of nerve growth that will lead to a cure for Alzheimer's Disease. He is furious with his professor, who doesn't seem sufficiently impressed. At times he doubts himself and feels insignificant, but at others he boasts about his creativity and complains that others are jealous of him. In turn, he is jealous of students who seem to be advancing faster.

He quickly becomes infatuated with women, gets very involved, then just as quickly feels they are disappointing and moves on to the next conquest. Those around him find his self-promotion and shallow relationships tiresome.

The social cost of these various mental and emotional illnesses is unknown, although it is clearly very great. In terms of the health care system, the people with these problems not only seek help from mental health services, but they go to family doctors and other medical specialists with physical complaints. Since treatment too often has only short-term results, these people can get into a cycle of crises involving other people, resulting in anxiety, depression and self-destructive behavior.

The disorders appear to be relatively common — one review estimates six to 10 percent of the population suffers from problems of this type, with the cases equally divided between the sexes. But since there are no strict criteria for exactly who should be counted as being "sick," these estimates are not entirely helpful.

Only recently have there been systematic, scientific attempts to categorize these disorders. From 1975 to 1985, the number of publications in this field tripled, and the *Journal of Personality Disorders* began publication in 1987.

However, there is still a long way to go. Until there is general agreement on the classifications, it's impossible to study causative factors, the natural history of the disorders, and what works best for whom. Given the mix and match nature of human personality traits, solving these problems is not an easy task.

*** Treatment

There are no set treatment formulas for personality disorders. The whole psychiatric tool kit — drugs, psychoanalysis, behavior therapy, group therapy, community therapy — has been tried by someone at some point, but not in the controlled studies that would prove which one, or which combination, is efficacious in each particular situation. Fortunately, much more formal studies are now being carried out.

One fundamental problem in this field is that there are not good data on the outcome for these people if they are not treated. Of course such data are necessary to develop any scientific analysis of alternative treatments and to determine whether treatment makes any difference in the long run. Some of these people do go on to more serious illnesses; most of them do not.

One American study reported that only 54 percent of the patients with borderline personality disorders who began treatment continued for more than six months, and only one-third completed it. Of these, a mere 10 percent were considered by their therapists to have been successfully treated.

There is some evidence that relatively short-term supportive therapy, aimed at improving coping skills and reducing behavior that interferes with everyday objectives, may at least reduce their use of health services, self-destructive behavior and problems at work. As well, there is some indication that this therapy may work better in groups, where patients can encourage each other to acknowledge the traits which cause many of their problems, like blaming others, impulsiveness and self-defeating patterns.

*** Research

There's a one-word answer to where research is needed with regard to these disorders — everywhere.

Specifically the questions are:

- What are these problems?
- Who tends to develop them and why?
- What are the effects on their children?
- Since most treatments are relatively ineffective, should they be withheld until something better comes along?
- Who does benefit from what, and why?

Psychiatrists who have had a great deal of experience with these people think some aspects of personality disorders are related to inborn features like temperament — their degree of emotionality, orderliness, gregariousness. A child may be predisposed to difficulties if his environment does not allow him to express these traits, or learn to control them appropriately.

It is also generally accepted that early childhood experiences may be important. Repeated sexual abuse in childhood is often reported by those with borderline personality disorder, and, as one would suspect, the severity of the abuse seems to correspond with the severity of the disorder.

Narcissistic people often had a lack of early admiration, and may be making up for this by now seeking an excessive amount of it. The boredom and emptiness they feel may reflect a lack of emotional responsiveness, as if they have been brought up in an emotional vacuum.

What is needed is systematic, coordinated scientific research that generates facts, instead of the observations, impressions and opinions that have dominated this field for so many years.

Chapter 6

Addictions

Addiction is one of those terms that everyone uses, but few can define with scientific accuracy. It's especially common to hear it used in contexts which do not involve disease, such as "chocoholic" for a person who thinks a fun evening is eating Black Forest cake with chocolate milk chasers.

Definitions of this term can be as casual as "alcoholism is drinking more than your doctor does," or as generalized as the World Health Organization's:

> *Chemical addiction exists when the chemical use has begun to interfere with the physical, psychological, social, occupational or domestic functions of the patient.*

Substance misuse, abuse, dependence and addiction mean different things to different people, but the common thread with all of them is that the person's use of a substance is creating problems. Abuse is generally defined as behavior that results in impairment of social or occupational functioning, and has produced psychological or physical problems that have lasted for at least a month.

Strictly speaking, addiction has the additional feature of "tolerance," where more of the substance is required to get the same effect. Also involved is "withdrawal," where certain other symptoms appear when the person reduces use of the drug. Those symptoms vary with the substance in question.

The Diagnostic Statistical Manual of Mental Disorders, a psychiatrist's bible published by the American Psychiatric Association, did not actually define addiction in its latest revised edition, but it did specify diagnostic criteria for dependence and abuse. At least three of the following behaviors constitute dependence when they have persisted for at least a month, or have occurred repeatedly over a longer period of time:

- the substance is often taken in larger amounts or over a longer period of time than the person intended;
- there is a persistent desire for one or more efforts to reduce or control consumption;
- significant time is spent in activities to obtain or take the substance, or recover from its effects;
- there are frequent intoxication or withdrawal symptoms when major work, school or home obligations need to be met, or when use is physically hazardous;
- social, occupational or recreational activities are reduced or abandoned because of substance use;
- use continues despite knowledge of a social, psychological or physical problem that is caused or worsened by the substance;
- tolerance has developed so that at least 50% more is needed for the desired effect;
- there are withdrawal symptoms when use is discontinued;
- the substance is often taken to relieve or avoid withdrawal symptoms.

"Abuse" is defined as continued usage despite knowledge of persistent or recurrent problems caused or worsened by the substance, and/or recurrent use in situations when such activity is physically hazardous, such as drinking and driving. Roughly 10 million Americans are regularly engaged in these types of seriously self-destructive behavior patterns.

Man's ingenuity in finding substances that will alter his mood or state of consciousness appears limitless, whether it is the ancient alcohol of fermented fruit, or the "designer drugs" of illicit laboratories, churned out in an alphabet soup of products for the street trade.

The use of these compounds and their abuse are fraught with societal, religious and cultural judgments which vary with time and place. Social use of alcohol is generally accepted in North America now, but was banned during Prohibition, and is illegal in Muslim countries, where the punishment includes long prison sentences. In many of these countries the penalty for selling illegal drugs is death.

The problems that substance abuse can cause are remarkably varied — physical, mental, occupational, financial, personal, family and legal. Their costs to society are enormous and far-reaching. There is the cost of treating the resultant physical illnesses, such as cirrhosis of the liver in alcoholics, lung cancer and blood vessel disease in smokers. Careless smoking is a major factor in fires which destroy lives and property. Illicit drug users often turn to crime to support their habits. About half of the 50,000 automobile accident deaths each year in North America are directly related to "drinking and driving." Alcohol is also involved in about half of North America's murders and suicides. Substance abuse is a major factor in reduced productivity and accidents in the workplace.

Alcohol, barbiturates, narcotics, sedatives, hypnotics and tobacco are the classes of substances most associated with physical dependence. From a biochemical viewpoint all of them except tobacco act as depressants on the central nervous system — they have effects similar to a general anesthetic.

There is still some scientific controversy regarding the true physical dependence of some of the abused stimulants, but some professionals in the addictions field consider cocaine a harder addiction to treat than heroin, especially when it is consumed in the form of "crack." However, many studies have shown that nicotine is the most addictive of all these substances.

In one study, rats given unlimited access to heroin for 30 days escalated their use in the first two weeks, then maintained a steady level, and remained in fairly good health. Those supplied with cocaine injected themselves until seizures or exhaustion prevented them from further use, but when they recovered, they went back to binging on it. After 30 days, two-thirds were dead.

Although cocaine is relatively new to the headlines, and has become a major North American drug problem, it is far from new. Sigmund Freud wrote about it and used it more than 100 years ago, and it was a common ingredient in many products, including Coca-Cola, until legislation banned it in the early 20th century.

What is new is "crack," a crystallized cocaine that can be smoked and is relatively cheap. It takes just eight seconds for its effects on the brain to peak, compared to several minutes for intravenous administration, and about an hour for cocaine taken orally. This fast effect, and the relatively short time until it wears off, is considered to be a major factor in its abuse: more must be taken quickly to maintain the desired effect.

When cocaine is taken through the nose (snorting) or intravenously, the average time from first use to complete addiction is about two years. With crack, an addictive pattern of use may be established within days.

Severe and potentially fatal effects can occur just as fast, sometimes with the first use, including seizures and heart attacks. Crack use is now the main cause of stroke in people under 30 in some major North American cities.

The exact causes of these strokes and heart attacks have not been fully researched, but since cocaine produces a fast and significant rise in heart rate, blood pressure, and body temperature, it is believed some of the deaths have their basis on pre-existing, symptomless structural abnormalities in blood vessels that could not withstand the stress of the drug.

Unlike other stimulants, cocaine depresses the respiratory system, and if it is combined with depressants like alcohol, to combat the insomnia and hyperactivity of cocaine use, there can be serious effects on the ability to breathe.

Cocaine's effects on the nervous system are centered in several of the chemical neurotransmitters that allow messages to race along from one nerve cell to another. These chemicals are excreted at the end of one cell, bridge the gap to the next cell and activate receptors there. The gap is normally cleared between messages; the leftover transmitter is reabsorbed and taken back to the first cell. But cocaine prevents this reabsorption, so the cells think more messages are coming and stay in a state of excitement. At the same time, the supply of the chemical transmitter is being depleted because it isn't being reabsorbed, and eventually the cells can't communicate. The drug is also a local anesthetic, and some scientists feel this effect on the central nervous system is a factor in the seizures it can provoke.

Unfortunately, the psychological effects that are pleasant in mild doses have a severe flip side with high doses or prolonged use — euphoria can become irritability, hostility and fear. Increased energy can become boundless energy leading to exhaustion. Postponement of sleep can progress to total insomnia. Reduced appetite can become complete loss of appetite — a weight loss of 30 pounds in the heavy user is not unusual. Increased feelings of self-esteem can become grandiose delusions, and an increased sexual drive can reverse to a complete loss of interest in sex.

Multi-drug abuse occurs in 30 to 70 percent of people with substance problems, in an infinite variety of combinations of alcohol, prescription and street drugs.

The effects of alcohol and drug abuse spread far beyond the person indulging in the self-destructive behavior. They can be devastating to the spouse and children, who are most directly involved with the abuser, and be transmitted to subsequent generations by the dreadful memories of their family experiences which children retain.

Margaret's father was an alcoholic whose drinking left the family so financially strapped she had to leave high school and get a job. Yet at 17, she, too, married an alcoholic and had five children in the next six years. She frequently felt depressed, and blamed it on hormonal imbalance after her pregnancies. She drank heavily during her last pregnancy, and was told her baby was neurologically sluggish after its birth.

The Children's Aid Society visited frequently after she returned home, but she wasn't drinking and was functioning fairly well, taking anti-depressants. Then everything fell apart when her husband came home drunk and abusive one night: she went on a drinking binge and didn't come home for four days. She continued with periodic binges, attributing her behavior to some medical disorder that hadn't been detected.

A particularly tragic group are the babies born addicted to, or damaged by, the substances taken by their mothers during pregnancy. Fetal alcohol syndrome, a group of defects caused by maternal drinking, is a major preventable cause of mental retardation in children, and is explained more fully in the chapter on retardation.

American surveys suggest that 10 percent of all babies are born to women abusing some chemical, and in some urban areas it is twice that, therefore roughly 365,000 babies a year are at risk. There is a long list of illicit and prescription drugs whose overuse can result in a baby undergoing withdrawal symptoms at birth including:

- morphine
- heroin
- methadone
- codeine
- amphetamines
- barbiturates
- tranquillizers
- alcohol
- phencyclidine (PCP)

These withdrawal symptoms include wakefulness, irritability, shakiness, diarrhea, excessive sweating, disorganized sucking, respiratory distress, and failure to gain weight. There is also an increased risk of prematurity, of growth retardation before birth, and of sudden infant death syndrome (SIDS), where seemingly normal babies are just found dead in their cribs, usually in the first year after birth.

The effects often live on through the child's development, with increased risk for hyperactivity, decreased school achievement, speech delays, poor motor coordination, perceptual difficulties, decreased attention span and behavioral problems. They are also more likely to become substance abusers themselves, and at an early age.

*** Causes

One standard book on addictions lists 43 theories of causation, and the scientific jury is still out on which ones are valid. Physical, psychological, cultural and social factors can play a complex role in the development of dependency.

There can be a hereditary component in some alcoholism but it isn't known just what is inherited. One theory is that there is an inborn difference in physical reactions to alcohol: that for some people it initially takes more alcohol to get any effect, so they tend to drink more than those in whom physical effects appear rapidly.

Babies born to alcoholics and adopted by non-drinkers have been shown to have an increased risk of alcoholism. Sons of alcoholics have a four-fold higher risk of the disease than the general population. The risk for daughters isn't that marked, but it's still higher than normal. Up to 50 percent of the fathers of alcoholics, 30 percent of their brothers, six percent of their mothers and three percent of their sisters will also have the disease.

A number of psychological factors have been suggested, but it's difficult to separate cause and effect in people who are already dependent. No specific "alcoholic or addictive personality" has yet been scientifically identified.

Among adolescents who abuse drugs, the main predictors of abuse are a feeling of distance from their families, misuse of chemicals by their families and friends, early use of alcohol and tobacco, disregard for rules, and lack of religious involvement.

Social and cultural factors such as availability and acceptability play a role. High levels of alcoholism are associated with cultures in which adult drunkenness is accepted. In cultures where drinking customs and rules are generally agreed upon, where moderate drinking is accepted and heavy drinking condemned, alcoholism rates are low. People brought up in non-drinking cultures are less likely to drink as adults, but those who do have a higher risk of getting into trouble with alcohol.

A short test called CAGE is frequently used as a predictor of alcoholism. If the person answers yes to any of its four questions, there may be a problem:

- Do you feel you ought to Cut down?
- Are you Annoyed by people criticizing your drinking?
- Do you feel Guilty about your drinking?
- Do you have an Eye-opener first thing in the morning?

Certain groups are considered at higher risk for problems with various substances. Adolescents who experiment with drugs because of peer pressure, curiosity, excitement or rebellion may go on to the point that they "do drugs to feel okay." Depressed and anxious people, isolated women at home, executives under stress, and the aged coping with retirement, bereavement and reduced independence, may start relying on alcohol and/or prescription drugs to relieve their distress.

Doctors and other health professionals and their families are another high risk group, and one factor is easy access to drugs. In addition, doctors can also contribute to dependency by inappropriate prescriptions for narcotics to manage pain, hypnotics for insomnia or tranquillizers for stress.

*** Treatment

To paraphrase the psychiatrist in the recent John Ritter movie *Skin Deep:* "The first step to curing all your problems, which stem from being an alcoholic, is to stop drinking."

The next step is to rid the body of the substances being abused, but this is the relatively easy part, although medical supervision to prevent serious effects of withdrawal, such as delirium tremens (DTs) with alcoholism, may be necessary. Judicious short-term use of medications like tranquillizers and anti-depressants can be helpful if care is taken not to swap one dependence for another.

Some heroin addicts benefit from a methadone maintenance program. It, too, is an addictive narcotic, but it can block the craving for heroin, and stop the frantic vicious cycle of finding the money to buy it, often by crime or prostitution, and finding someone who sells it.

Getting the person into initial treatment may be difficult — the idea of stopping the drug can be terrifying. For example, one of the major features of alcoholism is complete denial of the dependence. The alcoholic may insist he "can stop anytime," or lay the blame on others — "you would drive anyone to drink" — in efforts to avoid treatment.

A relatively recent method of breaking through this denial is "constructive confrontation," where those who care about the alcoholic present a firm and united front. They reaffirm that caring, document how they have been affected by the drinking, and insist on treatment. Employee assistance programs (EAPs) work on a similar principle, documenting how substance abuse has affected work performance, and offering the alternatives of treatment or job loss.

As in many other diseases, the earlier treatment starts, the better the prognosis. Only five percent of alcoholics are on skid row, and those who still have jobs and intact families can often be better motivated to begin treatment — they still have something to lose.

Management programs for substance abuse are as varied as the substances themselves, and often a combination of them shows the best results, since the person's whole living pattern must be altered for continued abstinence.

Residential programs in specialized facilities, or inpatient programs of several weeks in general or psychiatric hospitals, may be necessary for some. Day hospital or outpatient programs can include educational sessions, treatment of medical complications, group psychotherapy, nutrition counseling, retraining in social skills, vocational counseling and relaxation techniques.

Half-way houses and rehabilitation communities can often be useful in some stages of recovery, as a way to ease people back into society step by step. Often these can be the same centers which were discussed earlier in connection with schizophrenia.

However, over the last dozen years or so a number of specialized firms have set up residential living centers which focus on people, often young people, who have significant problems with drugs in particular, and behavioral problems in general. To provide some sense of how this marketplace has evolved, it is worthwhile to consider the interesting approach utilized in the material employed to market some of these centers, which are often quite viable economically due to the demand for their services, and the considerable success which they sometimes report in dealing with

Figure 6.1
Illustrative Ad from Substance Abuse Treatment Program

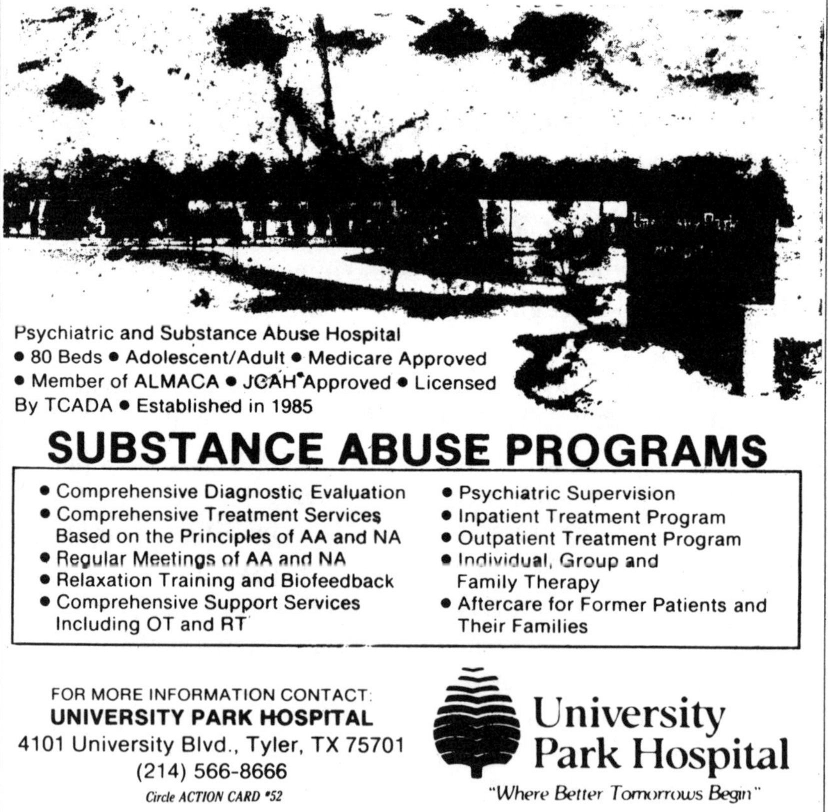

Figure 6.2
Representative Overview Marketing Material from a Large Scale Residential Treatment System

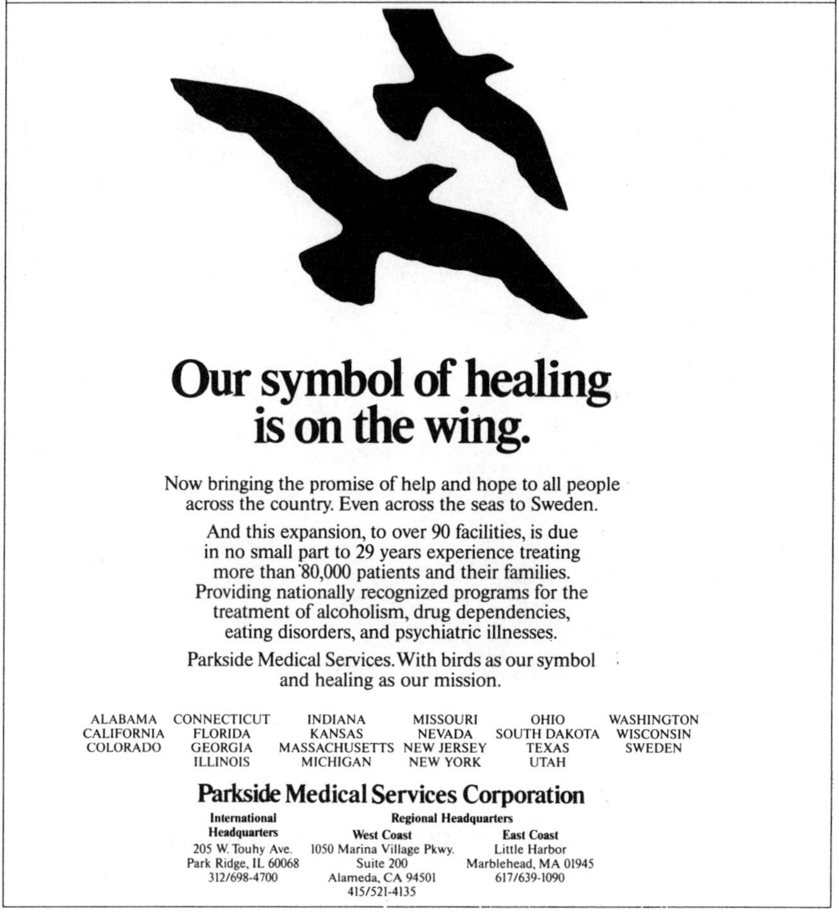

their patients. Sample ads are shown in Figures 6.1 to 6.2. A public sector program in Canada is pictured in Figure 6.3.

Family involvement is important, for everyone close to an addict is affected: they are often referred to as co-dependents. As well as needing education about substance dependence, they need to develop skills in breaking old patterns, such as indirectly sustaining the abuse by covering up or making excuses for it, and to restructure what have been chaotic relationships.

Almost one-third of substance abusers have major psychiat-

Figure 6.3
Front Building of the Donwood Public Sector Addiction Treatment Center Located in Suburban Toronto

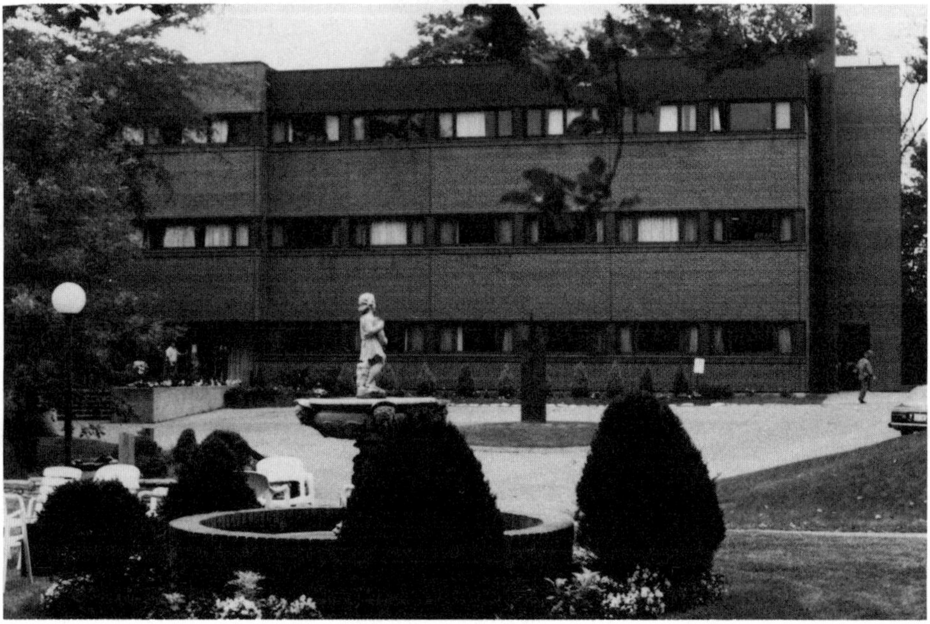

ric illnesses as causes or complications of their illness, and will require treatment for these.

Alcoholics Anonymous was the first self-help group devoted to a disease — it was formed more than 50 years ago in the United States, and has spread around the world, because it is successful, by emphasizing recognition of the problem, total abstinence, and a significant element of religious involvement. Since its first appearance in 1937, their flagship book, titled *Alcoholics Anonymous,* has sold approximately nine million copies worldwide. An international AA convention in Seattle held in the summer of 1990 drew over 45,000 people from all over the world.

Al-Anon and Alateen are also self-help groups for adults and teenagers closely involved with alcoholics, to help them understand and cope with the stresses in their lives. As a result of its success, AA has been used as model for Narcotics Anonymous and many other organizations.

Adult Children of Alcoholics is a more recent organization for those whose lives are still being influenced by their early experiences in an addictive family. This group especially helps people deal with the frequent reality that children of alcoholics often "act 40 when they are 14, and 14 when they are 40." The pressures to in effect take care of their parents' childish alcoholic behavior are great in their early years, and this often promotes a pattern of too-quick maturity, which seems to break down from time to time as they become adults. It has become clear that many of these people were virtually denied the normal period of relatively carefree childhood.

Communities vary in their formal programs and facilities for addiction, but family doctors, psychiatrists, clergy, mental health clinics, family service agencies and self-help groups can be sources of assistance.

These days, smoking cessation programs run a wide gamut: groups that meet weekly, day-by-day kits, acupuncture, hypnosis, and prescription nicotine chewing gum are just a few examples.

All of them work for some people, none of them works for everyone, and a smoker may have to try several before he or she finally quits. Although failure to quit may bring guilt and discouragement, studies indicate the more attempts a nicotine addict makes to quit, the better the chance for eventual success.

* * * Research

The past decade has seen a burgeoning of addiction research. Genetic studies have renewed investigations into the nature versus nurture combination, in order to delineate the roles of genetic compared to environmental factors.

Biological markers are being sought to detect which children of alcoholics are at particular risk for developing the disease, so preventive strategies could be aimed at them. New drugs are under investigation that would block the effect of alcohol at the cellular level, and stop the craving for a drink. As well, non-addictive drugs to reduce the severity of narcotic withdrawal symptoms are in the offing.

It isn't yet known why alcoholism, depression and antisocial personalities tend to cluster together in families. More studies are needed to determine which of the many therapies being used are most effective with which groups of abusers.

Preventive education programs for children which help them to deal with peer pressure, develop a healthy self-esteem and a life-style whose "highs" don't involve chemicals, have shown a great deal of promise, but require further assessment and refinement.

* * * For Further Information

In the USA

Alcoholics Anonymous is listed in most telephone directories, or one can write to Box 459 Grand Central Station, NY, NY 10163.

Al-Anon Family Groups and Alateen, P.O. Box 862, Midtown Station, New York, NY 10018-0862.

Alcohol and Drug Problems Association of North America (A.D.P.A.), 1130 15th Street, N.W., Suite 204, Washington, DC 20005.

National Council on Alcoholism (N.C.A.), 12 West 21st St., New York, NY 10010.

National Institute on Alcohol Abuse and Alcoholism (N.I.A.A.A.), 5600 Fishers Lane, Rockville, MD 20852.

Association of Labor-Management Administrators and Consultants on Alcoholism (A.L.M.A.C.A.), 1800 North Kent Street, Suite 907, Arlington, VA 22209.

In Canada

Alcoholics Anonymous (AA), Al-Anon and Alateen groups are listed in the white pages of telephone books.

Treatment, educational and self-help facilities vary widely among provinces and communities, but more information about each can be obtained from provincial agencies.

Alcohol and Drug Dependency Commission of Newfoundland and Labrador, 120 Torbay Road, St. John's Newfoundland, A1A 2G8. Phone: 709-737-3600.

Addiction Services of Prince Edward Island, Department of Health and Social Service, Eric Found Bldg., 65 McGill Ave., Charlottetown, P.E.I., CIA 7K2. Phone: 902- 892-4265.

Nova Scotia Commission on Drug Dependency, Suite 314, Lord Nelson Bldg., 5674 Spring Garden Road, Halifax, N.S., B3J 1H1. Phone: 902-424-4270.

Alcoholism and Drug Dependency Commission of New Brunswick, 3rd Floor, Victoria Health Center, Woodstock Road, Fredericton, N.B., E3B 5H1. Phone: 506-453-2136.

Chef du service des toxicomanies, Ministeres de la sante and des services sociaux, 1075 chemin Ste-Foy, 8ieme etage, Quebec City, G1S 2M1. Phone: 418-643-9887.

Addiction Research Foundation of Ontario, 33 Russell St., Toronto, Ontario, M5S 2S1. Phone: 416-595-6048. The foundation also publishes the 1988 Directory of Alcohol and Drug Treatment Resources in Ontario, with 350 entries: Marketing Services, Dept. OR, 416-6059.

Alcoholism Foundation of Manitoba, 1031 Portage Ave., Winnipeg, Man., R3G OR8. Phone: 204-786-3831.

Saskatchewan Alcohol and Drug Abuse Commission, 3475 Albert St., Regina, Sask., S4S 6X6. Phone: 306-787-4093.

Alberta Alcoholism and Drug Abuse Commission, 7th Floor, Pacific Plaza, 10909 Jasper Ave., Edmonton, Alta., T5J 3M9. Phone: 403-427-2837.

Alcohol and Drug Program, Ministry of Health, 1515 Blanshard St., Victoria, B.C., V8W 3C8. Phone: 604-387-4778.

Alcohol and Drug Services, Yukon Department of Health and Human Resources, 6118 - 6th Ave., Box 2703, Whitehorse, Yukon, Y1A 2C6. Phone: 403-667-5777.

Alcohol, Drug and Community Mental Health Services, Department of Social Services, Government of the Northwest Territories, 4th Floor, Precambrian Bldg., Yellowknife, NWT, X1A 2L9. Phone: 403-873-7904.

Chapter 7

AIDS

Inclusion of AIDS in a book on mental illness may seem strange, but this devastating disease is having a major impact on the mental health of millions. Since its recognition in the early 1980s, acquired immune deficiency syndrome (AIDS) has had a profound effect on society. It has dredged up comparisons with some of the most feared conditions in medical history, like plagues and leprosy, and the reactions have not been too dissimilar to those of our ancestors when they were faced with threats for which there was no known prevention or cure.

This widespread fear is taking its toll not only on the sick, but the well. In a remarkably short time by research standards, the human immunodeficiency virus (HIV) was identified as the causative agent for AIDS, perhaps in conjunction with other factors. It has also been determined that this virus isn't easily caught, like cold and flu viruses, by shaking hands or being in the path of a sneeze. However, the virus mutates and is apparently evolving, and some researchers are concerned that it will evolve to where it can be spread much more easily, perhaps even some day like a cold. Unlikely though it is, such a development, given our current knowledge of how to treat this disease, might mean the end of human civilization. At a minimum it would probably force all AIDS patients to be segregated from society.

Fortunately, at present the virus is passed on only through the exchange of infected blood and/or semen in sexual activity, through use of blood or blood products that carry the virus, through sharing contaminated hypodermic needles and syringes, and from infected mothers to their newborn babies.

The effect of AIDS on the body is devastating, and so far it is always fatal. A crucial component of the body's immune defence system is one type of white blood cell or lymphocyte, called a T- cell because the thymus is involved in its production. The HIV destroys a particular sub-type of T-cell, which is called a helper cell because it helps another type of lymphocyte to kill harmful invaders. The command center of the defence system is crippled, leaving the body open to what are called opportunistic infections from bacteria, viruses, parasites, and fungi; and to the spread of cancer cells. All these can become established like dandelions in an untended lawn.

Although treatments exist for most of these particular illnesses, each recurrence of them tends to make the body that much weaker until it is finally overwhelmed.

People with AIDS are bound to have severe mental repercussions. Not only are they facing death, but they may lose their income, friends, families — everything they cherish in life.

At the same time, the virus may directly attack cells in the nervous system in the same way it attacks T-cells. This physical damage, combined with the nervous system effects of the various infections and cancers that develop, and the multiple drugs needed to treat them, add up to profound neurological symptoms in half of AIDS patients at some time during their illness. At autopsy, neurological abnormalities will be found in 80 percent of AIDS patients.

When the disease has attacked the brain, people with AIDS may show signs that mimic mental illness even before symptoms of the actual immune deficiency manifest themselves: depression, delirium, dementia, personality changes, and episodes that resemble schizophrenia. There may be more subtle symptoms, like impairment of language and movement. In some cities with the highest rates of AIDS, it is now the most common cause of presenile dementia.

A person may view an illness as threat, loss, punishment, gain, relief or challenge. The psychological response to any major illness depends on many factors: how sick the person feels, what treatment is involved, his personality traits and coping skills, his support system involving other people, and how society views this particular disease.

Another group of people have a milder form of immune deficiency called AIDS-related complex (ARC), which usually involves swollen glands, and may include symptoms like fever, fatigue and weight loss. They may or may not go on to develop full-blown AIDS — no one knows how to predict which ones will — and this uncertainty brings a heavy emotional burden.

An even larger group also lives under a special burden of stress and uncertainty. They are the people who have been exposed to the virus and are assumed to be able to pass it to someone else. Evidence of their exposure can be detected by a blood test, but it can take months after their exposure for that evidence to appear, and no one can tell them whether they will develop AIDS or ARC.

So far, the majority have not developed either disease, but scientists cannot say with any certainty that there is a cut-off point after which the person won't get the disease. Our experience with AIDS and ARC is still too new for that.

The distress felt by all three of these groups tends to take four forms, with individual variations. Sadness, guilt, helplessness and suicidal feelings predominate when a person experiences a loss, whether it be loss of health, status, function, relationship or autonomy. Anxiety is produced by threats of loss or of stigma, or by threats to identity. Anger at one's self, at friends, family, or the helping professions is common. Withdrawal and social isolation may be self-imposed or forced on the person. Anger, fear and uncertainty are expected in these three groups, but they are also affecting many people who are not in the high-risk categories for exposure to the virus.

"AIDS has replaced cancer as the disease of choice among the worried well," is the way one AIDS support group spokesman puts it.

These are people who have an irrational fear of getting the virus in public swimming pools or saunas, from restaurant dishes and food, or from shaking hands with someone with AIDS. They have developed a plague mentality in the same way our ancestors huddled in fear against vengeful gods, or evils in the air.

In African countries, the disease is equally divided between men and women, and heterosexual sexual intercourse is the prime method of transmission. Unfortunately, partly due to the relatively informal approach to sexual activity in many of these countries, combined with poor health care facilities, and an almost total unwillingness to use condoms, it is presently estimated that a substantial percent of the population of all Africans will be infected with AIDS by 1995. In one such country, roughly 60% of the recruits for the army tested HIV positive. Certainly the situation in Africa is of epidemic proportions.

In the Western world, however, the majority of identified cases have been among two groups who were already treated with disdain by many in mainstream society — homosexual and bisexual men, and injected drug users. That fostered an "us" and "them" attitude that not only delayed the appropriation of government funds for research, treatment and education, but spawned such suggestions as isolation and quarantine of everyone with a positive HIV test, and the attitude that "AIDS is God's punishment for homosexuality."

With greater attention to "safe sex" practices in gay communities, such as wearing condoms and limiting the number of sexual partners, the focus of new AIDS cases in North America has shifted very rapidly to intravenous drug users who share needles, their sexual partners of either gender, and their infants. For better or worse, these individuals tend to live in poor areas of major cities. In the United States, abandoned AIDS babies have become a huge problem for some big-city hospitals.

Europe is facing this problem as well. For example, in one park in Zurich, authorities give away some 8,000 needles every day to drug users, in an effort to prevent the spread of AIDS and other diseases such as hepatitis.

Relatively small numbers of people have become infected through medical procedures. They received blood transfusions, or they were hemophiliacs with an inherited lack of blood clotting factor, and regularly used this factor extracted from the pooled blood of hundreds of donors. The availability of tests to screen donated blood for HIV has almost eliminated this danger in the western world. However, because of dreadfully inadequate medical facilities, most of the AIDS cases in the Soviet Union and Eastern Bloc countries are directly due to treatments received in hospitals. These generally involve the reuse of scarce medical supplies, especially needles.

*** *Treatment*

Since there is no cure for AIDS, medical care centers on the treatment of the individual infections as they occur, and general measures such as proper diet, exercise and sleep to help the body battle them.

Prolonged life expectancy has been shown in some studies involving the drug zidovudine, formerly called azidothymidine or AZT. It is no longer considered an experimental drug for AIDS, but it is still considered experimental for those infected with HIV who haven't yet developed the disease. Tests are underway to see if it can stave off the development of AIDS, but this use is controversial. Some argue that its early use may lessen its effectiveness if AIDS does develop, and its serious side effects cannot be justified in those who are not sick.

There is also a realistic economic consideration, since it costs thousands of dollars a year to treat one person with AZT, and there are many more people who are HIV-positive than there are people with AIDS.

Some people with AIDS are taking experimental drugs which attack the HIV, or prevent it from replicating, or boost the immune system.

Psychiatric treatment can be directed to the four stages that have been noted following the diagnosis of AIDS. Again, there are individual differences, and a person may go through one stage more than once.

- Denial is often a way of coping with overwhelming distress, and as long as it isn't carried to the extreme of refusing all medical care, it can be a protective mechanism for an initial period.

- In the next stage, denial is replaced by waves of sadness, anger, anxiety and guilt. They can be turned inward, with self-recrimination and thoughts of suicide, or outward, lashing out at others.

- In the third stage, there is a gradual acceptance of limitations and a new identity as someone with a life-threatening illness. Energy may be channelled into finishing a life's work, community services, or resolving difficulties in relationships with others.

- The final stage is a preparation for death. For some, the fear of dependency on others and loss of autonomy is greater than the fear of death itself. Suicide is frequently considered, but not often tried.

Supportive counseling and therapy, either individual or group, can help in devising strategies to deal with uncertainties, the wide range of emotions, the practical problems and relationship difficulties with partners, family, friends and co-workers.

Most major cities have AIDS groups with support networks of peer counselors, as well as therapy groups run by professional resource persons. Here, the person with AIDS can not only find help to alleviate the isolation he feels, but can learn from others who are in the same situation.

Medications such as anxiolytics (drugs to combat anxiety), anti-depressants, stimulants and anti-psychotics can play a practical role in relieving emotional symptoms and psychotic episodes, but they must be prescribed with particular care regarding both dosage and methods of action. The neurological damage that the disease or its treatment may have caused can create an increased sensitivity to side effects.

People who have a morbid fear of getting AIDS include those who are in a risk group but are healthy, as well as those who are at little or no risk. These feelings may persist in spite of their doctor's reassurance that there is no laboratory or other evidence to indicate that they are infected. Some of these people may have a mental disorder such as depression, panic disorder or hypochondriasis (an unrealistic belief one has an illness or disease). Others may be plagued by guilt, such as a heterosexual man who once hired a prostitute, or a married man who once had sex with a homosexual, and now fear AIDS as retribution.

No studies have proven that one type of therapy is any better than another in dealing with AIDS-related emotional problems, but various methods of altering thinking and behavioral patterns may relieve the symptoms. Short-term use of anxiolytics and antidepressants may be indicated in some selected patients.

Another group that may develop psychological problems related to AIDS is health care providers, even though their risk of getting the disease from patients is small if proper precautions are taken. The relatively few such cases that have been reported have usually involved accidentally sticking themselves with needles used to draw blood from AIDS patients. Education about the true risks, and strict adherence to infection prevention practices, are the prime methods of alleviating their concerns.

Burnout is another possibility among those caring for AIDS patients. These caregivers are often in short supply, and they have the additional emotional burden of having no cure to offer dying patients who are often quite young.

Prevention of burnout by awareness of its possibility and supportive programs for those at risk for it is easier than curing it.

*** Research

Massive research efforts have been mounted against AIDS in a relatively short time. They range from a greater understanding of the basic mechanisms of the immune system to devising the most effective methods of public education.

With no cure available yet, prevention is a major goal. Better methods of communicating the facts about AIDS to school children and the general public are needed to control the rumor mills that cause both unnecessary fears and unwarranted optimism that "it can't happen to me." More effective ways of getting general acceptance of safer sex practices, such as limiting the number of sexual partners and using condoms, are being explored.

In some jurisdictions, AIDS education programs have been mandatory in both elementary and high schools. Some high schools now have condom-dispensing machines, something which in most North American communities would have been unthinkable even 15 years ago.

Free hypodermic needles are being exchanged for used ones in some cities in the U.S. and Canada to cut down on the sharing of these items. Small bottles of household bleach to sterilize needles and syringes are also being distributed, but there are conflicting reports of the effectiveness of these measures in reducing HIV infection among drug injectors.

About two dozen potential vaccines to protect against AIDS are in some stage of development around the world, but there are formidable problems in such research and a proven vaccine is not expected to be developed, tested, and made available to the medical community much before the turn of the century.

Unfortunately, research has been considerably hampered by the fact that there is no good animal model on which to test a potential vaccine. Although some monkeys are infected by HIV, they don't get AIDS, so it's hard to tell if an experimental vaccine is actually protective. Researchers in several countries are trying to reproduce the virus in smaller laboratory animals, such as rabbits.

Successful vaccines usually contain a killed or weakened form of the virus which they are designed to prevent, and that poses unusual problems with HIV. It infects some of the cells in the immune system that must be activated to provide protection, and there are some fears that a vaccine might actually do more harm than good.

There is also a time factor. Because the virus can lie dormant for years, how will it be known if a vaccine is truly protective?

Ethical problems in vaccine testing also abound. For example, the best way of assessing effectiveness would be trials in a population where HIV is widespread. But these populations are mostly in developing countries, whose people might feel they were being used as guinea pigs by the more economically developed societies.

Around the world, scientists are working on medications

that will hopefully kill or deactivate HIV once it is in the body, or boost and protect the immune system.

In psychiatry, studies to show which techniques are most effective in alleviating the emotional impact of AIDS might lessen the huge psychological burden this disease brings.

* * * For Further Information

The following list is primarily devoted to general information. Many cities, provinces and states have AIDS hotlines, and information about services in local areas can be obtained from public health departments.

The Federal Center for AIDS, Health Protection Branch, Health and Welfare Canada, 301 Elgin Street, Ottawa, Ontario, K1A 0L2. Telephone 613-957-1772. FAX 613-954-5414. Coordinating Center for the entire federal AIDS program.

The Canadian Public Health Association AIDS Education and Awareness Program, 1565 Carling Ave., Ottawa, Ontario, K1Z 8R1. Telephone 613-725-3769. FAX 613-725-9826. Publishes an AIDS newsletter, The New Facts of Life. Includes the National AIDS Clearing House which collects and circulates a comprehensive selection of AIDS educational material from all over the world.

The Canadian AIDS Society/la Societe canadienne du SIDA. Box 3390, Station D, Ottawa, Ontario K1P 6H8. A national, non-profit umbrella organization for community-based AIDS organizations.

Helpful Organizations in the U.S.A

American Foundation for AIDS Research (AmFAR), 5900 Wilshire Blvd., 2nd Floor — East Satellite, Los Angeles, CA 90036; (213) 857-5900; and 40 West 57th Street, Suite 406, New York, NY 10019; (212) 333-3118

National AIDS Network, 1012 14th Street NW, Suite 601, Washington, DC 20005; (202) 347-0390

Both organizations publish directories of AIDS organizations, health care facilities and educational materials.

Helpful Organizations in Canada

AIDS Vancouver Island, 1175 Cook Street, #108, Victoria, B.C. V8V 4A1; (604) 384-2366 / 384-4554

AIDS Vancouver, 1033 Davie Street, #509, Vancouver, B.C. V6E 1M7; (604) 687-5220/687-2437

Vancouver PWA Coalition, P.O. Box 136, 1215 Davie Street, Vancouver, B.C. V6E 1N4; (604) 683-3381

AIDS Network of Edmonton Society, 10704 - 108 Street, Edmonton, Alberta T5H 3A3; (403) 424-4767/429-2437

AIDS Calgary Awareness Association, 1021-10 Avenue S.W. #300, Calgary, Alberta T2R 0B7; (403) 228-0198/228-0155

AIDS Saskatoon, P.O. Box 4062, Saskatchewan S7K 4E3; (306) 242-5005

AIDS Regina, P.O. Box 432, Regina, Saskatchewan S4P 3A2; (306) 525-0902

Village Clinic/Winnipeg AIDS Advocacy Council, P.O. Box 3175, Winnipeg, Manitoba R3C 4E6; (204) 453-0045/453-2114

AIDS Committee of Thunder Bay, P.O. Box 3586, Thunder Bay, Ontario P7B 6E2; (807) 345-1516

AIDS Committee of Ottawa/le Comite du SIDA d'Ottawa, P.O. Box 3390, Station D, Ottawa, Ontario K1P 6H8

Kingston AIDS Project, P.O. Box 2154, Kingston, Ontario K7L 5J9; (613) 545-1414/549-1232

AIDS Committee of Toronto, P.O. Box 55, Station F, Toronto, Ontario M4Y 2L4; (416) 926-0063/926-1626

Toronto PWA Foundation, P.O. Box 1065, Station Q, Toronto, Ontario M4T 2P2; (416) 925-7112

Safe Sex Project, P.O. Box 1143, Station F, Toronto, Ontario M4Y 2J8

Hamilton AIDS Network for Dialogue and Support, P.O. Box 146, Station A, Hamilton, Ontario L8N 3A2 ; (416) 528-0854

AIDS Committee of Cambridge, Kitchener, Waterloo and Area, P.O. Box 1925, Kitchener, Ontario N2G 3R4; (519) 576-2127

AIDS Committee of Regional Niagara, P.O. Box 61, St. Catharines, Ontario L2R 6R4

AIDS Committee of London, 649 Colborne Street, London, Ontario N6A 3Z2; 519) 434-8160

AIDS Committee of Windsor, P.O. Box 7002, Windsor, Ontario N9C 3Y6; (519) 973-0222/258-2437

Comite SIDA Aide Montreal, C.P. 98, Succursale N, Montreal, Quebec H2X 3M2; (514) 282-9888

Montreal AIDS Resource Centre (MARC/ARMS), C.P. 11; 64, Succursale H, Montreal, Quebec H3G 2N1; (514) 937-7596

Mouvement d'information et d'entraide pour la lutte contre le SIDA a Quebec (MIELS Quebec), 910 Avenue Brown, Quebec, Quebec G1F 2Z8; (418) 687-3032

Metro Area Committee on AIDS (MACAIDS), P.O. Box 1013, Station M, Halifax, Nova Scotia B3J 2X1; 902) 425-4882

SIDAIDS Nouveau Brunswick, Victoria Health Centre, 65 Brunswick Street, Fredericton, New Brunswick E3B 1G5; (506) 459-7518

Newfoundland and Labrador AIDS Association, P.O. Box 1364, Station C, St. John's, Newfoundland A1C 5N; (709) 739-7975

Books and Reports

Grieg, D. (1988). *AIDS: What Every Responsible Canadian Should Know*, Second Edition.Co-published by the Canadian Public Health Association and Summerhill Press. Available in English and French.

AIDS: A Perspective for Canadians, Summary Report and Recommendations. (1988). The Royal Society of Canada, 344 Wellington St., Ottawa, Ontario. K1A 0N4.

Langone, John. *AIDS: The Facts.* New York: Little Brown & Co.

Martelli, Leonard J., et al. *When Someone You Know Has AIDS: A Practical Guide.* New York: Crown Publishers.

Moffati, Betty Clare, et al. *AIDS: A Self Care Manual*, IBS Press.

Shilts, Randy. (1987). *And the Band Played On: Politics, People and the AIDS Epidemic*. New York: Penguin Books.

Spurgeon, David. *Understanding AIDS: A Canadian Strategy.* Toronto: Key Porter Books.

Chapter 8

Alzheimer's Disease

Fifteen years ago, if you stopped 10 people on the street and asked them if they could describe Alzheimer's Disease, chances are you'd have got 10 blank stares — or perhaps some wild guesses.

Today, it's estimated that up to 300,000 Canadians and at least 2.5 million Americans over the age of 65 have this disease. A recent study at a major Boston hospital has suggested that 10% of those over 65 have this disorder, and that this figure rises to 50% for those over 85. This new interpretation of the evidence would mean that the U.S.A. has about 4 million victims. Even with the lower figures, the disease accounts for about half the occupancy of beds in long-care institutions in North America, and is the fourth leading cause of death among people over 65.

This tragic disease gradually and inexorably destroys brain cells and nerve endings, taking with it memory, skills, personality, and all intellectual capacity. Death usually occurs within 10 years.

It can be heartbreaking for those who watch its progress, like the 70-year-old wife who had at first accepted the explanations of her husband, aged 75, that his forgetfulness was part of normal aging. He often couldn't find his car in the parking lot, or couldn't remember the name of his best friend.

But it got worse and sometimes dangerous. He would leave the stove burner on all night. He could no longer keep the monthly household accounts as he had done ever since their marriage. When he threw several family valuables in the garbage because he no longer remembered who they belonged to, or their value, she took him to the hospital.

The diagnosis of Alzheimer's Disease was made when other causes of dementia, such as brain tumor and small strokes, were ruled out. His name was put on a waiting list for a nursing home, and in the meantime he returned home, where his condition deteriorated steadily over the next six months, until he didn't even have control of his bladder while he slept. By the time he was in a nursing home for six months, he no longer recognized his wife when she visited, and one year later, he died.

This is no sudden scourge that, like AIDS, seemed to appear out of nowhere. It was described as far back as 1907 by Alois Alzheimer, a German neurologist who discovered distinctively tangled nerve cell fibers in the brains of some people who had died of dementia. But our delay in achieving a general recognition and diagnosis of Alzheimer's Disease was due to the mistaken idea that losing your mind was a natural part of the aging process. Indeed, senility, which simply means "old age," is still often used in general conversation to described loss of mental capacity: "Grandma's getting senile" is the explanation when she can no longer remember the names of her children, her address, or whether she had lunch today.

Alzheimer's Disease is not the only dementia (from the Latin for "without mind") of old age, but it is the most common, accounting for about 60 percent of the currently recognized cases.

Half of the remaining dementia is caused by multiple small strokes that cause scars and cysts within the brain. This multi-infarct dementia can occur even without arteriosclerosis, or hardening of the arteries. The other 20% of dementia cases are considered due to a mixture of degenerative and blood vessel diseases, or caused by conditions such as Parkinson's Disease.

There is also the possibility now that AIDS will become a major cause of dementia among the young in the future, because of its ability to destroy brain cells.

It is estimated that 1.25 million Canadians and 12 million Americans over 65 have dementias severe enough to cause some impairment in their ability to live independently.

At the onset of any memory loss, it is vitally important that depression is ruled out as a cause, otherwise elderly people may be institutionalized unnecessarily. They could be suffering from a disorder called pseudodementia, in which memory loss disappears with treatment.

In most of these cases, conversation and events don't get filed in the victims' memory banks. Such a person may not know what day it is, or where he is, or what he was told by a relative the day before. On the surface, this memory loss often looks like Alzheimer's Disease. The person may also be neglecting personal grooming, and may have lost weight. If he or she is elderly and depressed, there may be a shakiness and shuffling instead of a normal walk.

All of these symptoms, however, may be part of depression, in which thinking has become slow and labored, and problem-solving as well as behavior are now generally inefficient. It is strongly suspected that depression slows down the speed with which the front parts of the brain take up and burn glucose, the sugar in the blood which is their main fuel. With Alzheimer's Disease, brain cells are actually destroyed. In pseudodementia, by contrast, they are merely working less efficiently. When depression is treated with anti-depressants, these memory problems stop, presumably at the same time as the brain cells' ability to metabolize glucose returns to normal.

A minor form of the same problem can sometimes be seen in someone who is bereaved. An older person who has lost a spouse may appear to be losing his or her grasp of memory. This process may be part of the normal grieving process, which shares many features with depression, but is intermittent and gets better spontaneously.

*** Causes

The cause of Alzheimer's Disease is not yet known, although ten percent of all Alzheimer patients have a family history of it.

An increase in aluminum has been found in the brains of Alzheimer victims, but various studies failed to show a correlation to environmental exposure to the metal, such as cooking with aluminum pots. Small amounts of aluminum are present in a normal diet and can also enter the body through use of antacids and buffered painkillers, and from sprays and toiletries.

The aluminum theory came from work with experimental animals. After they were injected with the metal, microscopic tangles of nerve fibres could be detected. These looked the same as some of the degenerative changes found in cases of Alzheimer's Disease, but more recently, microscopic differences have been found in these two situations, somewhat discounting the aluminum theory.

Research continues on this controversial topic. A recent article in *Longevity Magazine* cites a study just completed at the University of Vermont College of Medicine, which found that rabbits injected with aluminum developed learning difficulties and suffered memory loss. The defects in brain chemistry and degeneration of the nerve cells discovered upon autopsy were virtually the same as those noted in Alzheimer victims.

On the other hand, people with severe kidney disease who must have waste products in the blood removed by dialysis machines may accumulate high amounts of aluminum, which results in some deterioration of nerve cells, but this damage doesn't look the same as that of Alzheimer's Disease under the microscope.

Overall, the consensus at present is that aluminum tends to accumulate as a secondary effect of aging or damaged neurons, rather than playing a primary role in the cause of dementia.

Alzheimer's Disease is not restricted to the elderly, although it is rare in middle age and extremely uncommon in those under the age of 40. The early onset form is called presenile Alzheimer's Disease, and for some unknown reason, it occurs two to three times as often in women as in men.

A recent discovery of differences in one area of the brain among Alzheimer patients may have pinpointed the specific location of the disorder. Information is transmitted along nerves with the assistance of chemicals called neurotransmitters. One of them, acetylcholine, is manufactured in the body of the nerve cells and travels to the end of the axons, or armlike projections. When an electrical impulse comes down the axon, a tiny drop of acetylcholine is released into the gap, or synapse, between its neuron and the next one, allowing the message to be passed on.

An important nucleus in the base of the brain, called the Nucleus Basalis of Meynert, has been found to be like a well of neuronal cell bodies that make acetylcholine, with axons that go to the cortex on the outer brain surface, which is the part that does the thinking and retains long-term memory. In the brains of Alzheimer patients, it has been found, remarkably, that there are 25% fewer of these cells in the nucleus.

*** Treatment

Since there is no known treatment that can prevent, reverse, or even retard the progression of the dementia, physicians can now only talk of managing the disease, and preventing its worst complications.

Alzheimer patients lose their judgment, so they can get into trouble in situations like turning on stoves or handling hazardous products in the home. While many will just quietly sit at home for hours on end, some have a tendency to wander, and can go out the door in freezing weather with few clothes on, or attempt to cross a busy highway without paying attention to traffic. The constant care and supervision they require is illustrated by the title of a book about caring for them. It's called "*The 36-Hour Day*."

The strain on the caregiver, usually a spouse, can be tremendous. The Alzheimer patient may become incontinent, get up frequently during the night, be unable to have a normal conversation, and develop a childlike dependence, wanting constant attention. There can also be frequent uncharacteristic outbursts of anger.

One wife described some of the results when she left her husband alone for brief periods while she did errands. He systematically ate all the contents of containers in the kitchen: flour, sugar, tea, spices. He took the front door off its hinges in midwinter, then lit the fireplace without opening the damper.

Greatly adding to the caregiver's burden is the knowledge that the situation will only get worse. To prevent his or her exhaustion and breakdown it is essential that community and other family resources be available for help. These can include day care centers for the Alzheimer patient so the caregiver can have some free time, relief care by someone who comes to the home for a few hours, support groups, visits by public health nurses, occupational therapists and community psychiatric nurses to provide advice and guidance, and temporary respite care so that the caregiver can have a vacation.

Remaining at home may preserve dignity and limit confusion for the person with Alzheimer's Disease. As the population ages, provision of services that will delay institutionalization as long as possible becomes even more essential from an economic point of view.

The Alzheimer Society of Canada estimates the disease is already costing $2.7 billion a year, and that it could affect up to one million Canadians by the end of the century. In a broader context, in the United States the National Institute on Aging estimates the cost of Alzheimer's Disease and dementias such as those caused by strokes, is about $90 billion per year. With the rapidly aging population, by the year 2050 there is expected to be 14 million victims of the disease, given current trends.

*** Research

Scientists have been hampered by a lack of an animal model for Alzheimer's Disease, and by the inability to directly study brain tissue in living patients. Indeed, the diagnosis of Alzheimer's Disease is only actually confirmed by examination of the brain after death.

Nevertheless, there are several active and hopeful research fronts.

In Alzheimer's Disease there is a clear lack of an enzyme essential for the manufacture of acetylcholine, important in transmitting messages among nerve cells. A whole range of substances has been tried to compensate for this deficit, and study results have often been accompanied by a fanfare of publicity about improvements, but the positive results have been short-lived. The search is still on.

The role of the tangles of nerve cell fibers, which are also found in Parkinson's Disease and the "punch drunk" syndrome, is also being examined. Genetic, environmental, immune system and possible viral factors are other research avenues currently being explored.

The nucleus of each human cell contains a complete blueprint for an adult human being, carried in 46 chromosomes, long chains of four different chemicals arranged in various sequences. The sequence determines the order in which amino acids, the basic building blocks, are linked together to form proteins. The chains are called DNA, and each segment of the chain that contains the instructions for one complete protein is called a gene — each chromosome has innumerable genes. Depending on the length of the chain, the number of genes could vary greatly.

When an abnormality in one chromosome is associated with a certain disease, that is the equivalent of saying the city in which the defect lies has been located. To identify the specific gene involved is like locating one house in that city, and then the particular chemical error that causes the defect must be identified.

Genetic studies have shown an interesting association between Alzheimer's Disease and Down's Syndrome, a genetic disease that has mental retardation as one of its features. By about 40, people with Down's Syndrome have changes in their brains that look like the tangled filaments and senile plaques found in Alzheimer patients. Down's Syndrome caused by an abnormality in chromosome number 21, and an abnormality in this chromosome was isolated in Alzheimer's Disease in 1986. But that doesn't mean the same gene is involved: the origins of the two diseases may be living in different houses.

The risk of having a Down's Syndrome child increases with the age of the mother. In a very interesting recent study, a similar association was shown between a mother's age and her child developing Alzheimer's Disease in later life, but this tentative result needs to be confirmed by additional research before being fully accepted.

Standardized methods of screening for dementias are needed. Fortunately, everyone who occasionally cannot remember where he put his car keys, or has to look up his own phone number, isn't a candidate. Better methods of measuring the degree and progress of impairment would also be helpful for assessing new treatments which may well be developed.

There are many tests of memory that can be simply applied, but these can be influenced by attentiveness, concentration, and distractions while the test is being conducted. New tests being developed would not be influenced by these factors. Such precise ways of testing would not only provide more accurate diagnosis, but would be valuable in assessing any new treatments designed to improve memory.

One new experimental drug has been found to increase metabolic activity in the brain area which is destroyed in Alzheimer's Disease. It remains to be seen if it produces real improvement in memory, but it appears to give a clue to the chemical that is needed.

*** For Further Information

Alzheimer Society of Canada, 491 Lawrence Ave. West, Suite 501, Toronto, Ontario, M5M 1C7. Telephone: 416-789-0530. It has many provincial and local chapters.

Guthrie, Donna. (1986). *Grandpa Doesn't Know It's Me*. New York: Human Sciences Press. (A book for children).

Powell, Lenore, and Courtice, Katie. *Alzheimer's Disease: A Guide for Families*. New York: Addison-Wesley Publishing Co.

Mace, Nancy, and Rabins, Peter. (1981). *The 36-Hour Day*. Baltimore: The Johns Hopkins University Press.

Chapter 9

Anorexia Nervosa and Bulimia: The Eating Disorders

In our modern western society, thin is in, and great numbers of people are counting calories or exercising to control their weight. But the victims of these two disorders go far beyond this.

The woman, and it's usually a woman, with anorexia nervosa may say she is aiming for an attractive figure, but even when she looks like the victim of famine she will insist that she is too fat. Many of these women literally starve themselves to death. It's not that they have no appetite or are disinterested in food: on the contrary, they are often obsessed with it. But they can't bring themselves to eat it.

> *Susan is a gaunt, 16-year-old high school student whose weight has dropped from 120, normal for her 5'7" height, to 95 pounds over the course of 11 months. She says she had felt chubby, and thought she'd be more attractive if she was thinner. She started by cutting out all carbohydrate-rich foods, then restricted her food even more, and started taking laxatives after she did eat. She has now become preoccupied with gourmet recipes and prepares them for the family, but doesn't eat them herself.*
>
> *She has little energy, has difficulty sleeping, and cries every day. Her menstrual periods have stopped. But she continues to be a conscientious and perfectionistic student and wins prizes for her high marks. Her parents have taken her to a doctor because*

they are so concerned about her weight loss, but she doesn't feel there is anything wrong with her.

People with bulimia also have a morbid fear of fatness, but they aren't as readily spotted by their body size: they may be under, over or normal weight because they both binge and "purge," i.e., frequently self-induce vomiting.

These people go into periodic feeding frenzies, wolfing down as much as 6,000 calories an hour, often in secret, so their families and friends are kept in the dark about their illness. One university student kept her roommates unaware of her binges by driving to a park at night with the front seat of her car loaded with junk food.

Often they follow such binges with purging to rid themselves of all those extra calories: they stick their fingers down their throats to make themselves vomit, take large doses of laxatives, and/or do a lot of exercising.

Anorexia nervosa affects about one percent of all North American women, and usually starts during adolescence. Bulimia nervosa affects less than one percent of women, and more may display some aspects of the two illnesses. Males account for perhaps only five percent of all cases of anorexia nervosa, and 10 percent of bulimia nervosa cases.

Both of these diseases have been recognized for centuries, although bulimia nervosa has only recently been described as a separate illness, and public awareness of these problems has only been widespread in the past decade or so.

The death of singer Karen Carpenter from anorexia nervosa not only publicized the disease, but reinforced its seriousness. Some observers attribute the dramatic increase in these disorders in the past 20 years at least in part to the influence of rail-thin entertainers and models — Twiggy was the extreme example.

We don't have any figures for the incidence of either disease when the Flemish artist Rubens was painting his ample ladies in the 17th century, but what was considered voluptuous then would certainly be labelled fat by most young western women today.

There is also some question as to how much of the increase in identified cases is due to a greater incidence, and how much to a greater recognition of the illnesses by doctors.

For the individual, unfortunately, neither of these illnesses tends to be a passing fad: they don't generally go away without treatment. They can continue for decades, if they don't kill first, and significantly impair all aspects of life, from work and health to relationships with others.

Estimates of the mortality rates vary, but as many as 10 to 15 percent of the sufferers of these illnesses die from their complications. Anorexics are more likely to die from the many secondary effects of prolonged starvation.

The purging measures taken by bulimics can derange their metabolic systems, depleting their bodies of potassium and causing abnormal heart rhythms and cardiac arrest. In addition, frequent vomiting exposes their teeth to the powerful hydrochloric acid in the stomach, and usually results in significant damage to their enamel, appearance and structural integrity. Victims of these diseases also have a higher risk of suicide.

*** Causes

It is generally believed that these problems start because of a psychological disturbance involving feelings of poor self esteem, helplessness and ineffectiveness. Limiting their food intake at first often gives anorexics a sense of being in control, but this does nothing to alleviate the underlying problems. In some cases, they must continue to diet to feel in control, and that leads either to starvation, or food binges and subsequent purging. They set up a vicious cycle. The emotional effects of their eating — or not eating — patterns lead to irritability, depressed mood and poor concentration. That makes their original psychological and physical problems worse, and they try, or in some cases, are driven to solve them by further dieting.

Unfortunately, they do not keep their illnesses to themselves. There is a higher rate of eating disorders among the children of parents with them, suggesting that at least part of the tendency to have them may be learned by example. Brothers and sisters of anorexics and bulimics also have a higher rate of the disorders, and recent research provides increasing evidence there may also be a genetic component.

*** Treatment

Help for these people must be at least two-pronged: correcting or limiting the physical damage done while establishing new eating patterns, and helping the person deal with the psychological and/or physical problems which set the whole cycle off in the first place.

Outpatient care is the first line of treatment, often in the form of a contract to maintain a certain weight in order to avoid hospitalization. Admission to a hospital for periods up to several months is recommended for the cases that require intensive monitoring of their food intake and nutritional status, and establishment of normal eating patterns. In rare cases, feeding through intravenous or naso-gastric tubes is required.

An outpatient hospital program may be beneficial in less severe cases. The patient attends daily for a few months, eats several meals, and takes part in a variety of therapies designed to improve her understanding of the illness, and to address the psychological disturbances that underlie it. Long-term ongoing aftercare is often necessary to resolve many of the family, interpersonal and social issues involved.

*** Research

The role of medications in these disorders is unclear: there is no "anti-anorexia" pill, although a few drugs can help with eating and weight gain. Some researchers claim that anti-depressants can bring dramatic results in bulimia; others do not achieve the same success.

New findings in brain chemistry and the systems that regulate feeding are pointing to new agents which may be useful, but much more research must be done on them before their safety and usefulness are established. Recent research suggests that one factor in bulimia may be a low level of serotonin, a chemical in the brain that sends out signals like "That's enough. You're full." For example, laboratory animals that are starving will not eat if their serotonin levels are artificially increased.

Many physical abnormalities accompany these disorders. Are they all effects, or could there be some biochemical or hormonal factor that is part of the cause?

While the need for psychological treatment is generally accepted, it is still unclear which elements of it produce changes in behavior, and whether it should be used in an individual or group setting.

More needs to be known about the role of the family. Is the illness genetic, environmental, or both? Is the family involved in the start or continuation of the illness, or both? If the family is involved in the onset of the disease, it might be possible to identify high-risk families, and work out strategies for prevention.

Factors which can predict the long-term outcome of eating disorders need to be understood, so that early targeted treatments can be applied to those at high risk for serious consequences. Also needed are effective ways to educate the public about the risks of inappropriate dieting, and the futility of trying to achieve some "ideal" body shape and size, while totally disregarding the realities of overwhelmingly important genetic factors.

*** *For Further Information*

National Eating Disorder Information Center, Toronto General Hospital, 200 Elizabeth St., 2-332, Toronto, Ontario, M5G 2C4. Phone: (416) 595-4156.

Chapter 10

Sexual Dysfunction

Including sexual dysfunction in a book on mental disorders would seem to lend credence to the idea that "it's all in your mind" if one has some problem regarding sexual function. But, perhaps nowhere else in human behavior is an artificial division between mind and body more inappropriate.

Our attitudes and behavior in expressing our sexual wants and desires are influenced by our upbringing, including the attitudes of our parents and the teaching of our religion, by the state of our physical health, and by our emotions and moods. But our ability to respond can also vary with the circumstances.

A woman who's put in a full day in the store, office or factory, made dinner, supervised the children's homework, and done three loads of laundry may be just too exhausted to welcome anything beyond some cuddling and caressing before she zonks out.

In the same way, a man who's been experiencing an unusual amount of stress at work, eats a big meal, and tops it off with a few drinks to "relax," may later also be unable to function sexually as he might wish.

These situations occur occasionally with everyone, and aren't considered sexual dysfunctions in the medical sense of the term. The old term "frigid" applied to women is no longer used, and the word "impotent" is applied for men only to describe a total inability to produce erections, even during sleep. They have been replaced with more accurate, and less pejorative descriptions. In women, the most common forms of dysfunction are:

- primary anorgasmia, where she's never had an orgasm with a partner;
- secondary anorgasmia, where she did have orgasms during lovemaking at one time, but no longer does;
- vaginismus, where the pelvic muscles go into an involuntary spasm, making it impossible for the penis to enter the vagina.

In men, the common dysfunctions include:

- primary erectile dysfunction, where he never did get an erection during sexual encounters with a partner;
- secondary, or situational erectile dysfunction, where he used to achieve erections, but no longer does, or fails to get them with certain sexual partners;
- so-called "premature ejaculation," when he has his orgasm long before he wants to: sometimes just by looking at his partner, at the merest touch of her, or immediately upon penetration.
- retarded ejaculation, the inability to ejaculate sperm, even with a firm erection and prolonged intercourse.

A syndrome known as lack of sexual interest has recently been added to the list of sexual dysfunctions.

Masturbation is not part of the list, because it isn't a sexual dysfunction, but a great many people worry about it. Although it is not damaging, aberrant or "perverted" behavior, many of the old myths live on. A century ago it was considered a cause of insanity, and about 50 years ago the Oxford Dictionary described it as "self-abuse." It definitely does not make you go blind or grow hair on your hands: if it did, our world would be full of guide dogs leading furry-fisted masters and mistresses.

*** Causes

Unfortunately, it is not as easy to explain the causes of these disorders as it is to list them. They often have several factors that impinge on one another. A therapist trying to assess a couple's problem will want to examine their total relationship, their attitudes towards sex, their knowledge of their own bodies and sexuality in its broadest sense, and any physical problems that may exist. In the latter category, for example, some drugs for high blood pressure or heart disease can interfere with the couple's usual activity.

Sexual response involves all kinds of body systems: blood vessels, nerves and glands, and therefore any illness which affects them can directly affect sexual function: diabetes, pituitary disease, multiple sclerosis, chronic kidney failure, cirrhosis or depression, to name just a few. Most sex therapists work in conjunction with physicians to sort out possible medical causes.

More indirectly, the stress or debilitating effects of an illness can also take their toll. "Not tonight, dear, I have a headache," is no joke to someone with a migraine.

Many people do not realize that alcohol is not a stimulant, it's a depressant, and large amounts of it have the same effect on sexual function as an anesthetic. Nor do many middle-aged couples realize that it normally takes longer to achieve an erection than it did at age 20.

"Fear of failure" can also play a role. The man mentioned early in this chapter, who couldn't develop an erection after a stressful day and a heavy meal, may not realize this is a temporary situation that can, and does, happen to everyone at some time. He may start worrying about it happening again the next time he tries to make love. He can develop so much anxiety about it that, in fact, it does happen.

When a couple is trying to conceive a child, and fails to do so after repeated and systematic attempts, sexual dysfunction can also result. Both partners experience the "fear of failure" under these circumstances. A woman who then resorts to artificial insemination in order to conceive can experience loss of sexual desire prior to or following the procedure.

Tensions in the couple's relationship can also play a strong role in sexual expression. Anger, resentment, frustration, and power struggles are hardly aphrodisiacs.

*** Treatment

A sex therapist is a professional with special training in the treatment of the disorders described above. He or she may be a medical doctor, psychologist, nurse, or social worker, for example, but whatever the original profession, special training in this field is essential.

Freudian psychoanalytical approaches were predominant for many years in the treatment of those sexual dysfunctions which were not easily attributed to some physical problem, but this technique has become much less popular over the last 20 years, due to changing views and knowledge of the realities about the nature, capabilities and roles of both men and women.

Masters and Johnson ushered in a new era of therapy after laboratory studies of humans led to publication of their book, *Human Sexual Response,* in 1966. They devised techniques for couples to take the pressure off performance in vaginal intercourse, to concentrate more on exploring sensuality in each other, communicating each other's likes and needs. Therapists now are turning to more of a smorgasbord of treatment. These can include debunking myths such as "the only real orgasm for a woman is a vaginal orgasm," or that a couple somehow fails if they don't have simultaneous orgasms.

The vaginal orgasm myth held that women should be able to reach a climax solely via "traditional" penetration into the vagina. It is now known that many women cannot have an orgasm by this method alone: stimulation of the clitoris is essential as part of the lovemaking.

Treatment can include education about how the body functions. It can explore problems other than sexual ones that may be getting in the way of sexual harmony. Adjustments can be made in certain medications, if they are a factor. Penile implants are sometimes suggested if the man is unable to achieve erections. Rods implanted in the penis come in a variety of designs, and the more recent ones can be bent for a more natural appearance when an erection is not wanted. Another design has hollow cylinders that can be inflated from a reservoir of fluid implanted under the skin in the groin area when an erection is wanted.

While they can be useful in some situations where there is a physical cause for erectile dysfunction, there are often other factors involved in the relationship, and a careful assessment of the total situation should be made before such surgery is undertaken. It shouldn't be seen as a "quick technical fix."

Many couples may find techniques other than vaginal/ penile intercourse equally satisfying. The only criterion is that it be acceptable and pleasurable to both partners.

While the range of recognized treatment techniques is wide, the field of sexual therapy can be open to abuses. In particular, it is never wide enough to accept any treatment method that involves the therapist becoming sexually involved with a patient, even on an intimate touching level. Patients encountering such behavior should run, not walk, to the nearest exit. Then report the therapist to his or her professional standards association to protect others from this unethical, and often dramatically detrimental, conduct.

Success of treatment often depends on who's evaluating it. Sometimes couples are quite happy with what the therapist considers as an insufficient resolution. "Cure" rates are also often based on results just after treatment, not on long-term follow-up.

But the willingness of both partners to devote considerable time and effort to therapy, and a caring, healthy relationship between them, is an important factor.

*** Research

One of the research challenges in this field is how to obtain valid assessments of the efficacy of various treatments: methods of obtaining, measuring and analyzing data. Ethical concerns play a big part in sex research, and there are important social concerns about answering questionnaires in survey research. A cautionary note: legitimate researchers absolutely never telephone people to do these surveys, but it's a common practice among people who get sexual gratification by asking intimate questions of strangers.

Also needed is research into the role that sex education programs may play in preventing sexual dysfunction later in life. The physical causes of impotence need more investigation, and the cause of persistent disappearance of sexual interest in people who are not depressed is poorly understood.

Unfortunately, we still have little understanding of any biological basis, if there is one, for sexual orientation and choice. For example, we do not understand why sexual interest sometimes becomes attached to unusual objects such as clothing, or why someone is stimulated by looking but not at all by touching.

*** For Further Information

The New Our Bodies, Ourselves. (1984). Boston Women's Collective. New York: Simon and Schuster.

Calderone, Mary, and Ramey, James. (1982). *Talking with Your Child About Sex*, New York: Random House.

Comfort, Alex. *The Joy of Sex*. (1972). New York: Brown Publishers.

Man's Body: An Owner's Manual. (1976). Diagram Group. New York: Paddington Press/Two Continents Publishing Group.

Chapter 11

Dangerous Sexual Practices and Sexual Anomalies

A society's acceptance of sexual practices and preferences can certainly vary with time and place. What was considered breathtakingly immoral between the covers of Playboy magazine 20 years ago is now routinely found on the cover of the supermarket checkout stand tabloids. But even in communities where there are no legal sanctions against a particular type of sexual behavior, some groups may still condemn it for deeply held religious reasons, or due to fears about the lowering of community standards, attracting unsavory strangers, and so on.

In general, as far as the law on sexual practice generally is concerned in North America, the rule of thumb is that anything two consenting adults do in private is their own business. But all three conditions are important: consenting, adults and privacy.

Nevertheless there are sexual practices which are universally condemned by law in the western world: incest, sexual abuse of children, and sexual assault, which has now replaced rape in the Criminal Code of Canada, and which includes lesser offenses than rape itself.

It has only been in the past few years that we have started to get an idea of the magnitude of these problems, particularly those that occur in the home. Even adult victims are often reluctant to report these crimes because of fear, humiliation, or a misplaced sense of guilt or shame.

In Canada, for example, the Badgley Report of 1984 estimated that more than half a million women across the country suffer some adverse effects on their health as a result of long-term psychological effects of sexual abuse in their childhood. These problems include suicidal behavior, poor self-image, inability to trust anyone or develop close relationships, guilt, anxiety, and depression.

In a California study of almost 1,000 randomly selected women, 38 percent claimed to have been victims of sexual abuse, including incest, before they were 18. In a Boston survey of both sexes 12 percent reported childhood sexual abuse.

Sexual offenders understandably do not usually confess to the full extent of their crimes, but a New York research team that guaranteed confidentiality and freedom from prosecution came up with some numbing figures after interviewing 232 child molesters whose victims were under 14 years old. Among them they had made 55,250 attempted and 38,722 completed molestations on 17,585 victims. On average, each had committed 170 actual molestations, and another 240 attempts on more than 70 children. The same researchers found that 89 rapists had raped, or tried to rape, an average of seven victims each.

But while the usual image of a rapist or a child molester is that of the stranger lurking in an alley, or the "dirty old man" hanging around schoolyards or parks, women and children are much more likely to be sexually assaulted by someone they know. It could be a parent, sibling, or more distant relatives, a baby sitter, or a friend of the parents. In particular, "date rape" is the term now used for situation when a woman is forced into sex by a man with whom she has gone out socially, but whose sexual advances she has refused.

Courts used to hold that a husband could not be convicted of the rape of his wife, even if they were separated or he used violence, but this is no longer the case. In addition, sanctions against sexual harassment and molestation, particularly in the workplace, have been included in quite a variety of the more recent human rights and labor legislation.

What seems like a new epidemic of sexual abuse within the family probably has more to do with recognition and reporting of such offenses, rather than an increased incidence of them. For much of this century, wives and children had few rights, and were generally considered a man's property. His home was his castle, and what went on within its walls was nobody else's business.

In particular, although it seems remarkable to us today, early psychotherapists took the same incredulous attitude as society about even the possibility of incest. Thus, when female patients told Sigmund Freud about childhood molestation by their fathers, he generally dismissed these discussions as little more than sexual fantasies. Not only were therapists unwilling to believe such things happened, but the patients were extremely unlikely to admit that they did, because of their intense shame and guilt, and the idea that somehow they must have been responsible.

*** Treatment

One of the biggest problems in treating the perpetrators of these crimes — who are most frequently men — is that they try to deny, rationalize or justify their behavior. Some of them just can't understand what all the fuss is about. Group and individual therapies are provided in most clinics and institutions dealing with sex offenders, but traditional psychoanalytic methods have for the most part been abandoned, because they were unfortunately proven to be ineffective. This is particularly interesting because many areas of medicine are under pressure to prove that they are effective, indeed that they are cost-effective, that is, worthwhile considering the costs involved, which are increasingly paid by insurance companies with many accountants. In contrast, here is a case where a medical technique was generally agreed to be not helpful.

In some areas of the world, castration, or removal of the testicles, is used in dealing with convicted sex offenders. This approach has never been widely used in North America, although many mayors have often heard about the merits of this treatment from shattered victims, and their hysterically angry relatives. Considering that surveys show 80% of Americans are enthusiastically in favor of the death penalty for murders, and traitors as well, it may not be long before the medical approach to sexual offenders is eclipsed in some areas by more direct methods.

On the other hand, drugs that block the effects of sex hormones and reduce sexual urges have had some success with these people, but of course those who might best benefit from these medications often refuse to take them.

In one recent study of 103 child molesters, only 45 were willing to admit even having a problem of sexual attraction towards children, and to undergo laboratory tests of sexual preference, or showed any interest in treatment. Of those 45, only 15 were prepared to participate in a three-month trial of Provera, a hormone to reduce sex drive, and eight of these people dropped out during the trial.

Behavioral modification techniques, with or without hormones, are also favored by some psychiatrists. A recent study of child molesters who agreed they had a problem generated a success rate of 70 percent after the end of treatment. These people were taught to have unpleasant fantasies when the sexual urge and thoughts of children's bodies surfaced in their minds. In addition, they were encouraged to masturbate frequently so that they would be sexually satisfied much of the time.

As might be suspected, many men with sexually deviant behavior have problems being assertive in acceptable ways, and often have major gaps in sexual knowledge. Fortunately, it has been shown that both of these problems can be corrected with assertiveness training and education. Despite the general failure of psychotherapy for severe sexual deviants, some men can be helped to develop better social skills, to make contact with more appropriate adult sexual partners, to express their needs and feelings in a more acceptable manner, and to reduce their general anxiety level. A part of this training is to help them learn how to fill the unstructured parts of their days, when their thoughts might otherwise drift into fantasies about their former preferences.

In the treatment of sexual dysfunction it is also important to deal with any co-existing psychiatric and physical illness which may be compounding the problem. Unfortunately, alcohol and other drug problems are often additional complicating factors with these unfortunate men, and treating these dimensions is also required to achieve any lasting results, and to stop them from developing illicit fantasies, or acting on them.

*** Other Sexual Anomalies

Psychiatrists use the general term "paraphilias" to refer to a group of disorders where intense sexual urges involve inanimate objects, children, non-consenting adults, or the induction of suffering in either partner. Sexual sadism, sexual masochism, and pedophilia (sexual preference for children) are the most serious of the illegal categories, and the most abhorred by society.

But other anomalies are criminal offenses. Exhibitionists publicly expose their genitals. Frotteurs get sexual gratification by rubbing against a strange woman's clothing or body in crowd situations. Voyeurs, or Peeping Toms, peer into windows to watch women undressing or couples in sexual situations. Interestingly, the statistics show that almost all of these behaviors are exclusive to men — we do not often hear of a Peeping Polly.

More than 30 types of paraphilia disorders have been listed by researchers, but most of these are rare, and some are not illegal. The fetishist, for example, who gets gratification from objects such as women's clothes or shoes, is in no trouble with the law unless he starts stealing garments from stores, off clotheslines, or from women themselves.

On the other hand, making obscene telephone calls can under some circumstances be illegal, and is certainly disapproved of by society in general. A famous recent case is that of the 51-year-old president of American University in Washington, D.C. Although very popular with students, faculty and alumni, he apparently made numerous obscene phone calls, particularly regarding children. When told by police that he was under investigation for these activities, he resigned, even though he was one of the most widely known people in Washington. For such an offense one can face criminal misdemeanor charges, which could involve a jail sentence of 12 months, and a $1,000 fine. He immediately enrolled in the Sexual Disorders Clinic of Johns Hopkins Hospital in Baltimore, where he underwent a course of therapy and counseling.

Scientists have recently determined that paraphiliacs often have a number of sexual deviations, and may unfortunately progress from one to another.

* * * Research

There are little solid scientific data about the origin of sexual anomalies, or which personal and environmental factors are important in their development. To solve these questions, scientists are exploring the complex relationship between sex hormone levels, the hypothalamus in the brain, and the sexual behavior of the individual.

Hormones secreted by the sex glands, the testes and the ovaries, are regulated by the brain, particularly the hypothalamus, a small unit at the base of the brain. It regulates many different chemical and hormonal functions in the body, including sexual behavior. But the role of the higher parts of the brain with regard to sexual activity is not yet well understood. Scientists are exploring, for example, how testosterone, the male sex hormone, feeds back into the brain from the bloodstream to elicit sexual arousal. They are examining brains by means of new imaging techniques, such as the PET scans mentioned earlier, to see whether the same parts of the brain are activated by hormones in normal people and those with sexual abnormalities. They are asking questions such as:

- What is missing from people who fail to regulate their sexual behavior?
- What brain mechanisms are involved in adult sexual behavior?
- What leads to pedophilia: is it simply a brain disorder or is there an overriding social component involving a severe lack of appropriate learning and development?

Of course, finding ways of reaching those who have eluded detection, or have not yet acted on their urges, might alter the disastrous course they are on, and would be of obvious benefit to their potential victims. Psychiatrists are heavily involved with this search, partly because of the criminal law implications of the behavior being investigated. With the rising public outcry against such conduct, and the admitted failure of many programs to either change or control people with these psychiatric problems, the legal system may increasingly step in where science has been unable to produce results. But such solutions tend to be punitive, expensive, and not at all aimed at solving the underlying problems. Even if they are actually imprisoned, some change in the behavior and attitudes of these people is warranted, because in almost all cases they are eventually, after enormous public expense, released into society again.

More generally, as in so many mental disorders, better ways are needed to help determine which individual people are likely to benefit from which particular treatments.

*** For Further Information

The New Our Bodies, Ourselves. (1984). Boston Women's Collective. New York: Simon and Schuster.

Calderone, Mary, and Ramey, James. (1982). *Talking with Your Child About Sex*, New York: Random House.

Comfort, Alex. (1972). *The Joy of Sex*. New York: Brown Publishers.

Man's Body: An Owner's Manual. (1976). Diagram Group. New York: Paddington Press/Two Continents Publishing Group.

Chapter 12

Emotional Disorders with Mental Retardation

Chicken and egg debates about which came first, or what is cause and what is effect, are common with mental disorders. In particular, with the mentally retarded it used to be generally assumed that if they displayed abnormal behavior it was part of their retardation: they repeatedly banged their heads against a wall, lashed out in anger at others, or remained mute because their brains were damaged.

It is now recognized that things are not quite so simple. Some of this behavior can be attributed to the original brain disorder. In fact, retarded people may have any of the psychiatric disorders in addition to mental retardation. Other disturbances may be a result of the effects that the retardation has had on relationships with others.

From early infancy, a mother may have trouble forming the usual bond with an infant who looks unusual, and is slow to respond to her. If there is inconsistent care, hostility, fear or even anger, the baby may become even slower in language and intellectual development. As a reaction, vomiting, frequent episodes of infection and diarrhea, head banging, blanket and finger sucking, rocking and sleep disturbances, can be part of the child's early distress, usually in the more severely retarded infant.

All this is in marked contrast to many mildly retarded babies who are described as very good, quiet children. When a child is late in walking, talking and becoming toilet trained, he doesn't develop the same sense of mastery and independence that toddlers usually achieve, and he can be set up for a lifelong sense of failure and low self-esteem. With adequate counseling, supportive and realistic parents who neither overprotect nor overstimulate can avoid many of these pitfalls.

That does not mean that parents are to blame if a mentally retarded child or adult also becomes mentally ill. They are no more immune to psychiatric disorders than anyone else in the general population. In fact, research has shown that they are several times more likely to have difficulties in adjustment, to experience more anxiety, and to show disturbed behavior more frequently than children of normal intelligence.

Given the defects in their central nervous systems, their developmental problems, and reduced ability to communicate, it is not unreasonable to expect that they will have greater difficulty dealing with the stressful situations we all experience, and be more prone to emotional and behavioral problems.

A fascinating study in the Isle of Wight in England found that mental retardation was associated with a five times greater prevalence of anxiety disorders, conduct disorders and adjustment reactions. If the children also had evidence of brain damage, the prevalence was actually six times higher. On the other hand, children who have physical characteristics associated with retardation, like those with Down's Syndrome, appear to have less trouble than those who look normal, perhaps because less is expected of them.

The term mental retardation covers a wide spectrum of disability, from those who cannot even control their basic bodily functions, to those who can live independently with some supervision. In general, over the past two decades there has been a swing away from housing even the more severely mentally retarded in vast institutions: more of them are living at home, as has been the case with the mildly retarded. More recently, they are also being integrated in regular school classes in some areas.

By the time a retarded child is physically and mentally ready to play, he may be older and bigger than the children who play at his level, and unable to keep up with the games of children his age. This may intensify his sense of inferiority, and inhibit him from trying new or competitive experiences.

Children with mild retardation may not be diagnosed until

they start school, and it is found that they can't keep up academically. In adolescence, when there is a strong need to identify with a group, to gain some independence from parents, and to make career choices, the child may become even more dependent on his parents, or react aggressively and display delinquent behavior.

But on the other hand, it is well known that older retarded individuals value conformity, and are more likely to be helpful and cooperative, rather than independent and competitive. Nevertheless, they are not immune to the same factors that produce criminal or antisocial behavior in the general population. Statistically, they are over-represented in criminal populations for petty crimes, but not major offenses. This could be due to the fact they aren't smart enough to avoid being caught, their greater likelihood of pleading guilty, or of confessing to a crime whether they committed it or not.

Especially in retarded people, unacceptable expressions of sexual urges may bring them into conflict with parents or the community. In the past, placement in an institution was often a result of homosexual behavior in boys, and promiscuity in mildly retarded girls, a punishment that would never have been tolerated for young people of normal intelligence indulging in the same behavior.

Involuntary sterilization was also a common practice, but civil rights legislation has sharply curtailed this approach, even though parents sometimes request it, particularly for girls. The idea that they would have babies more retarded than themselves, and that they would be unable to care for their children, was a motivation behind these measures.

Studies of successful marriages among mentally retarded adults have shown that when the parents had some outside help with child care, on average the intelligence of the children was close to normal, and higher than that of either parent. In addition, the parents had no higher incidence of child abuse or neglect. Nonetheless, this remains a controversial area due to social pressures, often from taxpayers who are in many cases struggling to raise their own families, even under completely "normal" circumstances.

*** Treatment

The same techniques of psychotherapy, behavioral therapy and medication available to those of normal intellect who have mental disorders such as depression, anxiety or schizophrenia can be useful with the mentally retarded, but often require some distinct modifications.

In an aggressive episode, where the safety of the person and others around him is in jeopardy, temporary isolation, a short-acting sedative, and personal restraint by physical holding may all be necessary. Mechanical restraint should always be a last resort. Aversive conditioning — a mild electric shock given when the person does something injurious to himself or others — is a controversial technique that is offensive to many people who read about it, especially in connection with the retarded. It is clearly a last resort and has been justified in some cases as a way of preventing serious injury. On the other hand, precisely this sort of conditioning is used by expensive private treatment centers to help people stop smoking, drinking, or using a wide variety of other drugs.

In one case, a young mentally retarded boy who repeatedly and compulsively banged himself on the head was causing quite a lot of personal injury. Even though he was given a protective helmet, the staff was concerned about the effects his severe pummeling might eventually have on his brain. Therefore he was given mild shocks each time he hit himself, and quickly learned to associate this self-destructive behavior with the pain of electricity. In a short time he stopped his compulsive actions, and needed very little subsequent therapeutic reinforcement of this kind.

A careful record of problem behavior and its various symptoms — their severity, the circumstances, and the frequency with which they occur — can be helpful to both the family and any therapist involved with sorting out the picture and establishing priorities. This background may provide the information needed to intervene in problems like temper tantrums, head-rolling, head-banging, rocking, and screaming.

Control of disturbed behavior through psychoactive drugs is common in the treatment of mentally retarded individuals. The smallest effective dose for the shortest period of time should be the rule for them, and drugs should be primarily for the patient's benefit, not that of those caring for them. As an example, it turns out that an effective medication in this area is depo provera, a birth control drug for females, which has been used in recent years for some males with sexually acting-out behavior, such as publicly masturbating several times a day. It works by directly reducing the production of the male hormone testosterone.

The excessive use of drugs for the treatment of anxiety, such as Valium, or antipsychotic drugs, like chlorpromazine, has led to controversy and the sense that these medications were being used strictly to control behavior. In contrast, many practitioners and researchers feel that patience, firmness and kindness might do just as well if they were dispensed properly. While psychotherapy was often avoided in the past because therapists didn't think the mentally retarded had sufficient ability to communicate verbally, many more are now having success with this approach.

Prevention is always preferable to treatment, and though it may seem incredible, maternal drinking during pregnancy is estimated to be the third leading cause of mental retardation in North America, after Down's Syndrome and defects in the neural tube early in pregnancy. As many as one-third of the babies born to chronic alcoholic mothers have what is termed fetal alcohol syndrome (FAS). It was identified in the early 1970s as a combination of physical, mental and growth abnormalities with lifelong consequences, although as far back as the Greek and Roman empires links were made between defective offspring and maternal alcoholism.

As illustrated in Figure 12.1, those with the full-bloom syndrome have a distinctive look — small heads, flat faces, small eyes set wide apart, short upturned noses, an underdeveloped upper lip and upper jaw, and facial asymmetry. They are small at birth, and never catch up to others their age. Heart, spine and joint defects, mental retardation, poor coordination and hyperactivity are common.

The severity of FAS seems to depend on the amount of alcohol consumed, but there are individual differences. Scientists have not yet established a safe drinking level during pregnancy,

Figure 12.1
Infant with Fetal Alcohol Syndrome

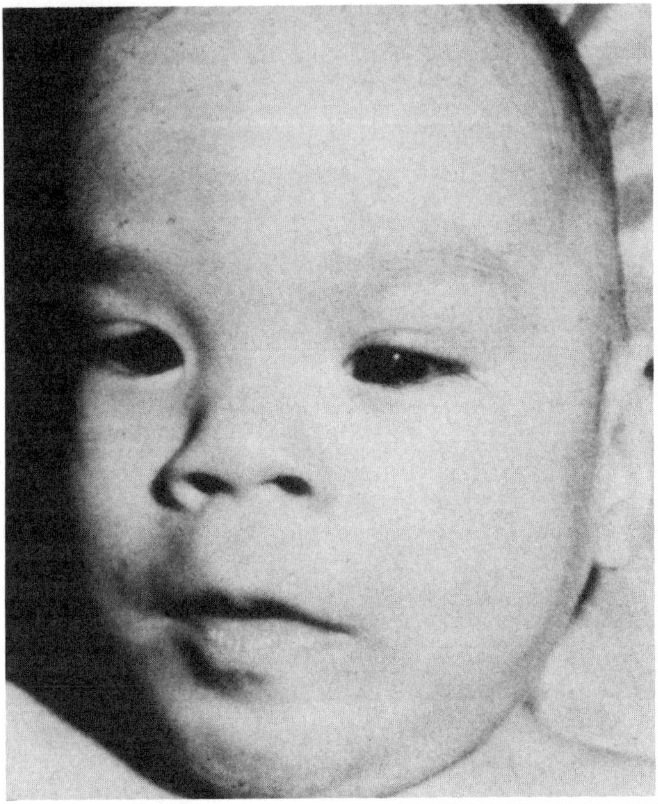

although many experts think there may be one, and doctors usually advise, "It's better for the baby if the mother doesn't drink."

*** Research

There have been major advances in understanding the causes and improving the treatment of mental retardation over the past 30 years, although this problem still directly affects one of every 100 North Americans. In particular, it is now possible to find hundreds of genes which lead to disturbances in brain chemistry which in turn can produce an intellectual handicap.

If these genes begin their action in infancy they produce mental retardation, as in phenylketonuria, where the child is missing an enzyme and will become retarded unless the situation is carefully diagnosed and the child is put on a special diet early in life. The absence of the enzyme prevents the breakdown of phenylalanine in the diet, which then accumulates in the blood, and can actually destroy brain tissue. This condition can be controlled by a special diet low in phenylalanine, for both the child, and during pregnancy in women known to have PKU.

When a defective gene's impact is expressed later in life, it can produce dementia or nervous system deterioration, such as in Huntington's Disease.

Research using modern biochemical techniques is vitally needed to determine the impact of these gene defects. Fortunately, it is now possible to find defects in DNA, the fundamental genetic blueprint, even before the associated chemical or enzyme effect begins.

The ability to diagnose hitherto unknown conditions is accelerating, and requires increased communication among scientists in the field. For example, the detection of Rett Syndrome, an autistic-like disease found only in girls, or Fragile-X syndrome, where there is a breakage of the X or female chromosome, was only possible after careful investigation of family pedigrees, and dramatic developments in analyzing tissues grown in laboratories. The difficult problems involved with Rett Syndrome and advice on how to cope with them have recently been explored in a first book on the subject, mentioned in the Reference section below.

A major advance in the field of mental retardation has been the development of more than 1,000 behavioral techniques to improve the ability of the mentally retarded to cope in society. But these diverse treatment approaches still require careful scientific analysis.

The biological revolution that led to drugs which can reduce the impact of schizophrenia and depression has only begun to affect the mentally retarded because of the difficulties involved in diagnosing these conditions in people who cannot verbally describe their symptoms. More careful and systematic approaches to such people with dual diagnoses are necessary.

A mother's exposure to the German measles virus during the first three months of pregnancy used to be a significant factor in mental retardation in infants before a rubella vaccine was developed. Now "cytomegalic inclusion virus" has become the number one infectious cause of retardation in newborns, striking one in every 1,000 babies, and a vaccine or treatment is sorely needed. The chemicals that cause a virus to reproduce can now be identified, and future research will probably succeed in finding a way to block the life cycle of the virus and stop the disease process.

In addition, new effective communications systems are urgently needed to overcome the language disabilities in mentally retarded persons, their biggest handicap after behavioral disturbances.

Chapter 13

Learning Disabilities

Whether they like it or not, school is a child's work.

It is an important part of the foundation for the rest of his life. Academic and social performance in the early school years can profoundly affect a child's sense of self-worth, and how his family, other children and adults perceive and react to him.

Learning, of course, does not begin with school. From early infancy a child begins to learn directly from his environment, examining his toes, shaking a rattle, identifying faces, exploring, touching, and of course eating everything. But it is school that puts a formal structure to learning. The child not only has to learn his ABC's, but he must do it in a setting where he can no longer talk or sing when he feels like it, wander off for a snack, or pursue whatever takes his fancy at the moment. And it is at school where learning disabilities are most likely to be first identified.

Under the broad definition of "an inability to keep up with classmates, or achieve academic standards considered appropriate for his intelligence," there are many kinds of learning disabilities.

Mental retardation, a lack of intellectual capacity, places limits on how much a child can achieve academically, but learning can also be impeded by alterations in the way a child's thinking influences his attention, concentration, memory and perception.

His incentive to learn can be hampered if those who are important to him don't seem to put much value on education, or if he gets little support or recognition from his family for his "work." For some children the effort required to achieve accept-

Table 13.1
Major Areas Affected by Learning Disabilities

Perception	Processing	Expression
auditory	memory	written
visual	organizing	verbal
kinesthetic	reasoning	non-verbal
spatial	evaluation	
temporal	extrapolation	

able "performance" may seem to be too much for the results they actually get, or previous failures may have led them to stop trying. Others are so disturbed by emotional problems and the energies they must exert in controlling anxiety or depression that they aren't alert enough to learn. Still others can develop neurotic problems, such as refusing to learn as a conscious or unconscious opposition to parents or teachers.

Personality conflicts with teachers, stress and problems caused by moves or changes of schools and teachers, absences due to illness, and other factors can all affect learning.

Certain types of specific learning disabilities have been identified in which defects or malfunctions make it extremely difficult for the child to master reading, spelling, writing and mathematics. It's not a lack of intelligence, although children with low IQs are not immune to it. Many of these children are very bright or accomplished in other areas of their lives. For example, Albert Einstein and Leonardo da Vinci both had dyslexia.

Joey, at 14, wasn't doing well in Grade 7, even though his mother was a teacher and spent a lot of time in the evenings tutoring him, and he had tested above-average on an intelligence test. He was good in sports, his health was good, and his hearing and vision were normal. In a Wide Range Achievement Test, he scored 10 on arithmetic, but only 5 each for reading and spelling, far below normal. When asked to read aloud, he substituted many words, generally choosing ones with appropriate meanings, such as "dot" for "spot," or "police" for " constable."

Dyslexia comes from the Greek for "difficulty with words,"

and to a dyslexic child, a printed page in English may just as well be in Greek. It is an inability to read, write and spell because written language doesn't make sense to the child. He is unable to make the connection between the written symbols and the words he uses every day in his speech.

He may be unable to distinguish between letters whose shapes are similar, but reversed, such as u and n, b and d, p and g. Words may also be reversed, so he reads was instead of saw, god instead of dog. He may be unable to distinguish between letters with roughly similar sounds, such as f and v.

Many of the dyslexic's spelling mistakes can be explained by the fact that he resorts to a homonym or phonetic equivalent—a spelling that sounds the same. So cough becomes kof or cof. But other errors are unexpected: celebrant for celebrate, or ginagtic for gigantic.

The dyslexic does not see words the way normal readers do, and in part this may be due to abnormal movements of his eyes: they stop in the middle of words, rather than between them. Consider the sentence below, which is broken at the points where one dyslexic's eyes were recorded stopping.

All th♦e anima♦ls at the zo♦o were loc♦ked in their c♦ages du♦ring

He may try to guess at a text: if he recognizes that a word starts with an "s," he may try a word he knows that starts with that sound, even though it is completely inappropriate.

Susan Hampshire, star of the TV series The Forsyte Saga, described how it felt to be a dyslexic child:

> *It is a lonely existence to be child with a disability no one can see or understand. You exasperate teachers, disappoint parents, and, worst of all, know no way of proving that you are not stupid. At school, I used to wait in terror for my teacher to point her finger at me and say, 'Susan, you stand up and read the next two paragraphs.' As I struggled to decipher the words, perspiration would roll down my arms and make little patches on the floor.*

Attempts at writing are just as disastrous: skipped words, syllables left out, jumbled spellings. The two figures below illustrate classic writing patterns characteristic of people with dyslexia:

Fig. 13.1: Fusion of two consecutive letters in the word "them"

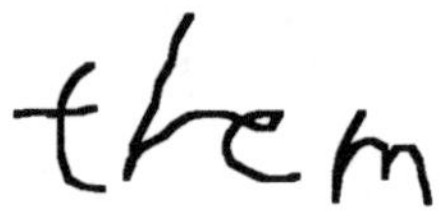

Fig. 13.2: Fusion and omission of letters in the word "basket"

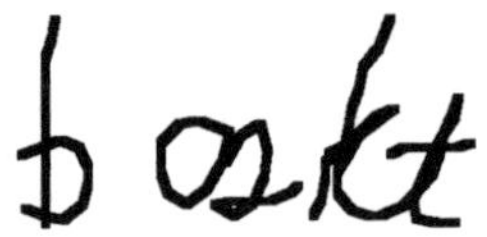

Another specific problem can be related to mathematics — the child cannot master the concepts of addition, subtraction, multiplication and division. Most of what we can say about arithmetic disorders comes from the study of brain-damaged adults, and it appears that the same kind of problems can occur in children without brain damage. While verbally fluent, and having a good verbal IQ, the performance IQ scale is relatively low. When given a mathematical problem, the child can calculate only at the simple rote memory level. If, for example, he has memorized multiplication tables, he might be able to calculate an answer that only needs this recall, but if the problem involved a new sum, he couldn't do it. Some children have both dyslexia and "nonverbal learning disability" or NLD.

Dyslexia is about four times as common in boys as girls, and may affect, to some degree, up to 10 percent of school children from all walks of life. Hyperactivity can also be associated with learning problems, and a separate chapter of this book is devoted to it.

But, no matter what the cause of the learning problem, the child may become maladjusted because of the poor self-esteem associated with repeated failure, and the way he is seen by others in his world.

Some parents may be unable to accept some imperfection in their children and openly or subtly reject him. Partly as a result, the youngster's sense of failure may lead to serious depression, and even suicide in some adolescents.

*** *What Can Be Done*

A thorough physical and psychological assessment is essential before a specific learning disability can be diagnosed, including hearing, vision, and any history of brain damage such as might occur if the mother was a heavy drinker during pregnancy, or after a difficult forceps delivery. In rare cases, young children have an infection which causes inflammation of the brain and may impair their ability to learn.

It is important to know if the child is emotionally distressed. Depression in children can be accompanied by a lack of motivation, pervasive sadness, poor self-esteem, a lack of confidence about learning, and a lack of curiosity to learn.

Intelligence needs to be assessed. Children with specific learning disabilities often have an IQ equivalent to that of normal children, but, like Joey, they might do poorly on tests of some specific subdivisions, such as verbal skills.

Learning-disabled children also have difficulty copying shapes, such as a triangle connected to a square. They seem unable to copy the line drawings in an orderly sequential fashion and are said to have a problem in perceptual motor functioning.

Family members perceive the child as having difficulty persevering at school and outside it. These children are seen as being anxious, poor at reading and spelling, and having a tendency to be clumsy. Their parents do not regard them as stable or well-organized.

Even when one learning disability is identified, like dyslexia, it doesn't mean that other problems such as emotional ones aren't affecting the child's ability to learn. A "global" approach to assessing all the factors in his environment is the best course.

A current theory of the development of learning disorders involves the manner in which the cerebral cortex, or specific regions of it, is organized. The arrangement of cells is determined during the middle trimester of pregnancy, when cells from the embryonic neural tube migrate out to the appropriate parts of the cerebral cortex. Errors can be made in the arrangement and sequence of the columns of cells that move out, through faulty instructions from genes, the mother's ingestion of a toxic chemical, or even possibly the production of a toxic chemical within the body.

These situations can lead to a cluster of cells not properly connected, or in the wrong order, producing an inability to perceive connections such as those between a sound and a set of letters.

It is recommended that students rehearse recognizing typical sounds or phonemes contained in words: it helps them learn to remember words, which they can do easily, and to recognize sounds that words have in common, such as she and he. Some students can't decode the written word and translate it into a sound, and they may need many rehearsals using different senses, such as listening to a tape of the text while reading it, or learning the shape and feel of a word by "sky writing" it, or tracing the letter to match the name of the object with its shape. After many rehearsals, the shape, feel and sound of the letters can often be firmly implanted in the student's memory.

Through spelling rehearsals the children can learn to locate words in the dictionary, eventually within 60 seconds or less. A daily instant spelling check reviews all the speech sounds already studied: the child repeats each sound, identifies it, names and writes the letter that represents it. In this way, he can learn to spell most words he needs without memorizing them as full words.

*** *Nonverbal Learning Disability (NLD)*

Some children with good intelligence have difficulty in learning arithmetic, but not reading and spelling. An intact left hemisphere is needed for verbal skills, and an intact right one for learning arithmetic symbols and other shapes, so it has been postulated that there might be some learning disability for spatial functions in the right half of the brain. It has now been discovered that those who have trouble learning arithmetic also have difficulty learning any kind of spatial configuration, and have coordination difficulties, particularly on the left side of the body, which is served by the right side of the brain. They may have some trouble writing because it's hard for them to learn the shapes of written letters.

Interest in exploring visual or tactile (touching) stimuli is minimal in these children, and they tend to be sedentary, rather than active. Speech tends to be rather flat and monotonous, because they lack the melody or emotional expressiveness of speaking that is a function of the right hemisphere.

People with NLD have trouble sizing up, organizing and synthesizing new and complex situations. They tend to rely too heavily on prosaic role behaviors which are inadequate, and as they age there is a marked tendency toward social withdrawal and increasing and dangerous isolation. In childhood, they tend to misbehave and are often labelled hyperactive. As they grow up, they often become underactive, and have excessive anxiety and depression, which gets worse with advancing years.

Remediation and rehabilitation for NLD children is crucial, but difficult. They give the impression that they are perfectly adequate because they read and spell well, but if their special needs are not met their futures may be quite bleak. For these people, spatial information, including shapes of written letters, has to be taught repetitively and with frequent and regular rehearsal. Any task that involves copying a shape should be accompanied by clear verbal instructions.

Youngsters with this disability also need to be taught to understand simple social situations at home and school so they can comprehend what is important and what is not; how to develop strategies to cope with specific problems; how to deal with ordinary gestures; and how to convey their feelings in a nonverbal way.

For learning disabilities in general, remedial instruction should primarily be provided in a school setting, but that doesn't mean parents shouldn't be actively involved. They also may benefit quite a bit from self-help groups.

Teachers are now more aware of learning disabilities, but

unless they have considerable experience, and a special interest in them, they alone cannot be responsible for a remedial program. They need the help of professionals in special education, psychology and mental health for a multi-dimensional assessment.

Ideally, every school should have access to someone with expertise in learning disabilities, either on staff or in the community. Such investments now can help save a fortune in later treatments as well as in social costs over many years in the future.

*** Research

There have been advances in understanding the underlying process involved with learning disabilities, but there still are few definitive answers for many concrete situations. Methods used to alleviate the problem may be limited to only one or two aspects of it, and our skills in this entire area need to be further developed and assessed.

Again, new brain imaging techniques such as PET scans offer a window through which brain function during learning can be seen. The task of learning to read, for example, can be broken down into its components to see which parts of the brain are involved in each step, and whether they have any subtle abnormalities. The next step would be to work out how to employ other parts of the brain: simultaneously reading and listening to the same words while the child is being examined by means of a scan or other related technology might be quite helpful.

*** *For Further Information*

Canadian Association for Children with Learning Disabilities, 323 Chapel St., Ottawa, Ont., KIN 7Z2. There are also division in each province.

Hornsby, B. (1984). *Overcoming Dyslexia*, Prentice-Hall Canada Ltd.

Chapter 14

Hyperactivity

This condition has had more names than Elizabeth Taylor in the last 30 years. Before 1960, it was called "minimal brain damage," but this became unacceptable because it could never be demonstrated there was some actual damage to the brain, nor was the problem minimal: these children were indeed having considerable trouble.

In the 1960s, it became "minimal brain dysfunction," to denote that there was some malfunctioning in the brain, rather than actual damage, at the physical or chemical level. Again, there was a problem with the word "minimal."

The next candidate was "developmental hyperactivity," suggesting some immaturity that the child would outgrow. This didn't hold up after long-term studies showed that half of children affected by this problem do not outgrow it, even in adulthood.

"Hyperactive child syndrome" is the term now in general use, although psychiatrists officially call it "attention deficit-hyperactive disorder," mercifully shortened to ADHD.

No matter how much the name changes, the picture is distressingly the same. These children, usually boys, are perpetual motion machines who can drive their parents crazy with exhaustion and frustration. From their earliest years they cannot seem to sit still for more than a minute. Their attention span is about the length of half of a TV commercial. They dash from one thing to another, rarely finishing anything. They are readily distractible by stimuli in the environment.

These youngsters aren't just overactive or unusually boisterous. Their activity differs from that of others their age in both quality and quantity:

- their impulsiveness results in sloppy work in spite of reasonable efforts
- they often intrude into or interrupt what others are doing or saying
- they have difficulty waiting their turn
- they get easily frustrated, which can lead to fights with other children

Even as babies, they may display more colic, sleep and feeding problems than normal infants. They may not enjoy being held for more than a few minutes, and this can be the start of a mother's frustration because she can't seem to comfort her baby.

As toddlers, they don't start walking, they start running. They may jump up and down in their cribs until they wear out the mattress, or climb over the sides. They have an unusual lack of fear, and require close supervision to prevent them from climbing into medicine chests or dashing into the street. Unfortunately, all too often their motto seems to be "late to bed and early to rise."

By the time he's about four the hyperactive child may be unable to play well by himself or with others. His quick frustration, lack of concentration and demanding ways quickly make him an unpopular playmate or guest.

Take him to someone's home, and he dashes from one thing to another, frequently breaking things, interrupting conversations and demanding attention. In addition, nursery schools may refuse to keep him.

His parents often complain that "nothing works," that neither praise nor punishment seems to have any effect. Some of them will respond to positive reinforcement that is more frequent, immediate and varied than that needed by normal children.

In elementary school, where concentration on studies and sitting for longer periods of time are expected, he not only becomes difficult for teachers to handle, but his achievements are below his intellectual ability. He fails, and then low self-esteem may be added to his other problems.

By the time he's in his teens, his most serious problems are likely to be school failure and antisocial behavior. A substantial number of these adolescents get referred to courts because of such things as truancy or theft. At a time of life when having close friends is so important, he may be unable to make them.

Hyperactive children have been reported all over the world, and in all types of settings, although prevalence rates vary widely. In some American cities, they are given as six in 100, while an incidence of one in 1,000 was reported for the Isle of Wight. These differences may be as much due to dissimilarities in diagnostic criteria and methods of collecting data as to actual differences in prevalence.

Even the ratio of five to nine hyperactive boys for each hyperactive girl has been called into question with the suggestion that boys are more often identified because they display more disruptive behavior. Hyperactive girls don't have any particular symptoms in contrast to the boys: they just display less of the same kind of behavior.

The causes of this hyperactive syndrome are unknown. As noted earlier, it used to be thought it was due to some type of brain damage, but this has never been demonstrated and the present trend is to suspect some type of brain dysfunction, possibly genetic in origin. We have some evidence that heredity factors also play a role.

There is widespread agreement, but not certainty, that an important factor here is an imbalance in the brain's system of catecholamines, chemicals transmitted down the arms or axons of cells and released at the nerve endings to bridge the gap between the next nerve cell. Norepinephrine is one such chemical, widely distributed in the brain and involved in alertness and attention, but there is evidence that one of its breakdown products, normetanephrine, is indeed higher in hyperactive children.

Giving D-amphetamine for two weeks will reduce the level of norepinephrine breakdown products in the urine. But despite this evidence, there is no conclusive proof of a disorder of catecholamine metabolism. Certain other drugs, such as amphetamines, which normally stimulate catecholamine activity, can work in a paradoxical way in the hyperactive child. One PET scan study of the effect of amphetamines showed a lowered metabolism in the area of brain controlling motor activity among hyperactive children, even though the drug speeded up this metabolism in normal youngsters.

It is well known that food additives and sugar have been blamed by some for aggravating hyperactive behavior, but carefully controlled studies have shown no conclusive association. Without their knowledge, but with their parents' permission, one group of children had been placed on a diet free of additives, while a comparable group ate food with normal additives, and their hyperactivity was measured by observers who didn't know which child was on which diet. Other studies have used a cross-over design — a child uses one diet for several weeks, then changes to another, and back again, with neither child nor parent knowing which diet contained additives.

Several such studies have reached the same result: food additives do not affect hyperactivity. Most doctors are convinced that this is probably true. However, some people cling to the opposite view, perhaps out of a need to believe there is some cause out there that is tangible and can be dealt with. This brings them a greater sense of security than the ambiguity of not knowing at all what the cause might be. In any case, removing or reducing the incredible quantities of these compounds which children eat probably can only help the child's health, in many ways.

Because psychiatrists are first and foremost physicians, from their point of view these additives, and "junk" food in general, have a disturbing dimension, in that the dosage of this material consumed is generally not related to the body weight of the patient involved. Indeed it often seems that there is an inverse correlation. When a "normal" nine-year-old boy consumes four purple Popsicles, two Cokes, and two bags of french fries in an all too typical afternoon, physicians can only lament that the dosage of sugar, artificial colors, saturated animal fat, and artificial flavors is colossal, relative to the perhaps 90 pounds of the child's bodyweight. The typical soft drink contains about 8 teaspoons of sugar, and as is well known the body converts sugar into energy when the pancreas produces insulin. Through a remarkably sophisticated regulatory system the pancreas tries to create and distribute enough insulin so that the level of sugar in the blood is just about always equal to 100 milligrams per deciliter, which amounts to only about 1 teaspoon of actual sugar throughout the entire body of a 155 pound person. Therefore when a physician sees a child eating a snack such as mentioned above, he can only see Johnny's poor pancreas jump on its bicycle and start pedaling furiously.

Fortunately there is no hard evidence to support the viewpoint that the excessive consumption of sugar, and other additives, actually causes specific physical illness. But of course diabetes is the disease which results when the pancreas gives up, or is destroyed by some unknown cause. Therefore, other things being equal, less consumption of these largely foreign additives will likely put less pressure on this and other bodily systems, compared to eating more of these substances, most of which generally did not even exist prior to World War II. In the context of the evolutionary experience of humans, many of these materials are relatively untested, compared to, say, spinach.

In any case, with hyperactive children it is difficult to separate cause and effect with regard to other important environmental factors, such as the family and school situations. At present, scientists cannot conclusively state how much of a child's behavior is a reaction to the way he is treated by his parents, teachers and peers, whose attitudes in turn are affected by the hyperactivity.

*** Treatment

Half a century ago, in a Rhode Island treatment center for children with disturbed behavior, it was found, somewhat paradoxically, that half of them showed improvement in behavior and school work if given stimulants. Methylphenidate (Ritalin), a synthetic medication having effects similar to amphetamines, now seems to be remarkably effective in about 90% of hyperactive children. Dextroamphetamine is another well tested option. Some youngsters respond better to one than the other.

Partly because of these results, the number of children

receiving stimulants under medically supervised conditions is increasing. One American study showed an increase from 1.1% in 1971 to 3.6% in 1983; another showed that between one and two percent of all elementary school children were receiving medication for hyperactivity.

Several well-controlled studies show that these medications apparently produce quite remarkable results. They evidently improve sustained attention, activity level, fine and gross motor performance, mathematical computations, memory, and relationships with others, while at the same time reducing impulsivity and aggression.

Nonetheless, there is concern among many parents and some mental health professionals that these drugs are being over-prescribed, although no surveys prove this. When this situation is suspected, the parent has every right to ask about the diagnostic criteria which were used to determine that stimulants were the appropriate therapy. It would be poor practice to give a child these drugs merely because he is aggressive or poorly behaved.

In fact, stimulants should only be prescribed on an individual basis after a careful assessment which includes a physical examination of the child, details about the pregnancy and the child's early development, the severity and frequency of any symptoms, the presence of any learning disabilities, and the child's views of himself, his family, peers and school. Interactions within the family and the school environment should certainly be included in this analysis.

A teacher skilled in coping with hyperactive children, and a remedial program that can be incorporated in the school curriculum may be an important part of any well thought-out plan, therefore if at all possible the teacher should certainly be invited to be part of any treatment team.

Considering that medical stimulants are often a helpful treatment, it may seem paradoxical that these children benefit most from a physical environment without excessive stimulation, and a clear and definite structure in the classroom to limit distraction.

Many hyperactive children require treatment other than, or in addition to, drugs. Training in social and self-regulatory skills, psychotherapy for poor self-esteem and any depressive symptoms, parent training, and even family counseling and marital therapy may be part of a tailor-made plan.

Unfortunately, even though medical stimulants can dramatically help deal with the hyperactive child's symptomatic behavior, they are not a cure. The results of several studies to look at the outcome of their long-term use have been disappointing, in terms of their effectiveness in actually solving the underlying problem. It may be that the children stopped taking the drugs regularly; the doses prescribed weren't optimal; they did not get the non-drug therapy they also required; perhaps they developed a tolerance for the stimulants; or these results may stem from a mixture of such factors.

Loss of appetite and sleeping problems are the most common side effects of the stimulants, and they can be alleviated by not taking the medication after mid-day. They can also trigger seizures in children prone to them, since they lower the seizure threshold.

There have been concerns that the stimulants can stunt growth, and some doctors stop them during the growth spurt that occurs in adolescence. It has been found that children grow normally by taking the drugs only on weekdays, avoiding them on weekends, and stopping their use completely in the summer time.

*** Research

The first priority is to devise diagnostic criteria that can objectively and reliably distinguish the disorder from over-activity which is merely due to excitement, lack of discipline, or other causes. This would do much to reduce uncertainty about who should be treated with drugs and other therapies.

The second priority is the discovery of a safer and more effective type of medication. Advances in the study of brain chemistry show promise in providing drugs tailored to hit their specific target, without undesirable side effects. Studies are also needed on the long-term effects of different doses of the stimulants now used with regard to their impact on academic, social and emotional adjustment.

There should also be a more scientific examination of the short and longer-term effects of different combinations of intervention programs for different sub-groups of children with ADHD.

In addition, existing educational techniques need to be improved to provide classroom environments, curricula, teaching strategies and behavioral management techniques better suited to the ADHD child.

Many studies are now being conducted on how to improve children's self-regulatory skills, an area central to this disorder, and although the techniques being developed look promising, they are not yet proven. It will be important to look at the way behavioral modification techniques and medications work interactively. Will the combined effect be better than the sum of the two given separately? Families would also benefit from more research on the most effective means for coping with these children. For the parents, any and all techniques which are shown to have scientific validity might be of immense importance for their peace of mind, but also for the sake of the siblings, peers and friends of the hyperactive child, who may be also severely affected by his behavior.

Chapter 15

Autism

An attractive little boy sits quietly, spinning the wheels of his toy car, ignoring everyone around him. An hour later, he's still spinning those wheels — not trying to push the car along the floor, not making "vroom, vroom" engine noises, just staring at the wheels going round and round.

He pays no attention to his mother's calls to come and eat lunch. He resists every attempt to take the car from him, and pulls abruptly away from his mother's efforts to get him to his feet. It is as if he is in a world of his own, one he wants neither to leave nor share.

The boy is not emotionally ill — he has autism, a brain developmental disorder that will affect his relationships with others for the rest of his life. It is the most severe of a group of conditions called "pervasive development disorders," or PDDs, which are related to the growth of the brain.

Autism is a syndrome, a collection of symptoms which together produce a complete lack of communication, lack of interaction, and resistance to even the smallest changes in routine. A child with this condition appears to have no interest in human attachments.

Autism has been called the childhood disorder with the highest burden of suffering for the families of its victims, and perhaps the worst prognosis for recovery. When first recognized, autism was thought to occur in four or five children in every 10,000, and four times more often in boys than girls. But in 1988, the largest and most comprehensive study of autism ever done in the world was carried out, among all children aged 6 to 15 in two areas of Nova Scotia. It came up with an occurrence rate of 11 to 13 per 10,000 — more than twice the rate previously assumed for this problem.

Most people might not even be aware of having seen an autistic child or adult. They have no distinctive physical appearance, wheelchairs or white canes. Symptoms among them vary considerably, and can be quite subtle in some cases. Those characteristics also change as they age.

Fortunately, this medical problem has recently gained a much higher profile from two fictional portrayals of autistics in recent years: Tommy, the son of Dr. Westphal in the TV series *St. Elsewhere*, and Raymond, the Oscar-winning role played by Dustin Hoffmann in *The Rain Man*.

As infants, victims of this problem may be described as "good babies," rarely fussing, and usually content to lie quietly in their cribs. But even at this stage there may be some signs of the trouble to come: poor sucking, lack of interest in people, sleeping problems. As the months go by the manifestations become more pronounced.

For example, autistic babies do not grin in recognition at familiar faces, and they can seem terrified by unfamiliar ones. They do not hold out their arms to be picked up, and they may stiffen at any attempt to cuddle them. They make no attempt to acknowledge their parents with "Dada" and "Mama," nor do they babble on in the nonsense syllables of babyhood. They may not even try to communicate by pointing at things they want. They can have an obsessive interest in certain toys or objects, like the little boy endlessly spinning his car wheels, but they don't play with them creatively. They don't even create an imaginary playmate to share their loneliness.

Autism in children is usually diagnosed in the toddler years, although these children may have reached kindergarten age before the disorder is fully recognized, depending on the severity of the symptoms in each case. In most cases, parents find their child's lack of responsiveness hard to accept. They are hurt by his resistance to any holding or cuddling, and feel rejected by his apparent message that he would be a lot happier if his world were not cluttered with other people. "Pat-a-cake" and "peek-a-boo" just do not interest him.

If he does speak, it may be only a constant repetition of everything that is said to him, or he may use words or phrases randomly and inappropriately. Equally difficult to deal with is his exasperating insistence that nothing should ever change. If his lunch is on a different plate, or his meat on a different side of it, an instant tantrum results. His socks must always go on the same foot first; he must always sit in the same place in the car.

These behavioral and developmental abnormalities make school years extremely difficult. His inability to appreciate the needs of others or alternative points of view may make other children see him as rude and selfish. He can't seem to carry on a normal conversation, or get the knack of listening to and following the conversations of others. He might memorize a whole bus schedule, and insist on reciting it no matter what anyone else is talking about. If he does make friends, they are likely to be younger children, or others with handicaps. His favorite TV channel might be the one that broadcasts nothing but weather, or perhaps the shopping channel.

Once he reaches his teens, he may want to be with others, but he easily becomes upset when he is not able to establish relationships with them. He has never learned the rules of the social game. He lacks the perspective to see himself as others do, and is probably unable to understand that they are laughing at him because he has said or done something which is generally regarded as silly or inappropriate.

If he manages to get a job which he can perform well, he might still be fired because of his odd behavior; for example, at coffee breaks one young man with this problem sat by himself, tearing up small bits of wet paper and sticking them all over his clothes. Another didn't know what to do with himself when his own work was finished, and aggressively tried to take over someone else's tasks.

About 75 percent of autistic children are also mentally retarded, although some have exceedingly high intelligence. About 30 percent develop epilepsy, usually in adolescence.

*** Causes

The possible causes of autism are unknown, and to make this situation more complicated there are indications that no two cases of autism may stem from exactly the same sources. There is evidence of physical and chemical abnormalities in the brains of these victims, and some disruption in very early brain structure or function, although research still has not determined how these fit together.

It used to be thought — and sometimes parents were told — that autism could be caused by severe emotional deprivation. This mistake only added unjustified guilt to the parent's already considerable emotional burden. There are tantalizing genetic elements in the as yet unexplained mystery of what causes autism. For example, this problem is more common among identical twins than fraternal ones. If one child is autistic, there is a slightly higher chance that a brother or sister will be. The fact that it is more common in boys than girls also suggests a genetic factor. However, in the rare instances where girls do have autism, it tends to be more severe than in boys.

There are many specific questions to be answered:

- what is the pattern of transmission of the disease
- what substances are or are not somehow transmitted
- exactly what proportion of cases have genetic origins

In addition, the roles played by complications during pregnancy and birth, which are common factors in autism, are not yet clear.

*** Treatment

There is no known cure for autism, and even though children do not usually outgrow it, they often improve dramatically as they age. Early and multifaceted help is essential for the development of maximum potential in the child, and to enable the parents to cope with the major stresses autism presents. To deal with the individual adequately may require the combined, closely coordinated, and ultimately very expensive, efforts of family doctors, psychologists, psychiatrists, social workers, speech therapists, educators and others with specialized skills.

Before school age, the treatment package should include medical and diagnostic programs, parent training and counseling, and pre-school programs for the child. The parents may also need specially trained baby-sitters, and respite care resources so they can take an occasional break from providing the continuing attention that such a child requires.

Fortunately, there is good evidence that these treatment programs work in reducing the negative impact of autism on the quality of the child's life, and in some children, they can have a major positive effect.

Formal education is also a challenge with these children. Everything from special classes to partial or full integration in regular classrooms has been tried to ensure a good education for autistic children — frankly the needs can vary dramatically with the child. But they also require leisure and recreational training and resources, pre-vocational and vocational assessment and training, and perhaps ultimately a place to live away from home.

Unfortunately, given our present limited abilities to deal with this severe problem, the multiple resources for employment, recreation, housing, medical care and continuing education will also be needed by those with autism into adulthood, and financial assistance may be required.

Low doses of drugs called neuroleptics, such as haloperidol and thioridazine, have been shown to be helpful in treating behavioral aspects of autism in some children, such as overactivity, self-injurious behavior like hand-biting or eye-gouging, aggression, repetitive behavior, insomnia and disorganization. However, these medications should not be taken for long periods without careful medical supervision and re-evaluation, because they can cause permanent involuntary movement disorders called "tardive dyskinesia," discussed in the chapter on schizophrenia.

Many other drugs have been tried, including Vitamin B6, magnesium, L-Dopa, and stimulants, but these have not proven effective, and so far the magic solution has not been found.

* * * Research

New technology developed to look at the structure and chemistry of the brain is bringing further insights into the causes of autism. The use of PET and MRI scans is still in its infancy in this field, but these technologies may prove valuable in detecting underlying differences in brain structure which contribute to this syndrome.

Currently, the latest research indicates evidence of an abnormal metabolism of dopamine, one of the substances that transmit messages in the brain. That may be why neuroleptic drugs can be helpful — they tend to work against dopamine.

Autism is also accompanied by a high level of another transmitter, serotonin, mentioned earlier in connection with suicide, and the importance of this chemical activity is being investigated. Efforts are being made to identify sub-groups of children with pervasive development disorders, to see which causal factors tend to point to which manifestations of the problems.

Of course finding a genetic factor and the chromosome on which it is located would be an enormous breakthrough in this field, and although research continues on this question, at present there are no especially hopeful results to report.

In addition to better understanding of the biochemical causes, it would also be helpful, on a daily coping basis, if we had far better methods of developing social skills in these children, modifying their behavior, and delivering education. Techniques to help in these areas would greatly improve the quality of their lives, and would also immensely assist the parents involved.

New medications would also be helpful. Lithium, a drug normally used to level out the hills and valleys of manic-depression, has been used successfully with a few autistic children who display episodic behavior at some times of the year, but studies continue to determine if this medication will be valuable.

Some researchers think that children with autism who injure themselves do so to release endorphins, the body's own opiates, and that medications which dampen the effects of these substances might be useful in curbing this behavior.

*** For Further Information

Autism Society of Canada, 20 College St., Suite 2, Toronto, Ontario, M5G 1K2. Phone 416-924-4189.

Grandin, Temple, and Scariano, Margaret M. (1986). *Emergence: Labelled Autistic*. Novato Calif.: Arena Press.

Wing, Dr. Lorna. (1985). *Autistic Children*. New York: Brunner/Mazel Publisher.

Chapter 16

Mental Disorders and Physical Illness

Complicated interactions exist between mental and physical health and illness, and sorting them out can become a chicken and egg exercise. For a given individual, which came first? These various problems may not even be related in terms of cause and effect. We certainly know that having a physical illness does not preclude you from getting a mental one, and vice versa.

Indeed, it is widely agreed that at least 20 percent of the people with a physical disorder also have a psychiatric one, even excluding alcohol and other drug abuse. Conversely, up to 40 percent of people diagnosed as having a psychiatric illness also have a diagnosable physical one, and in half of them, one illness seriously aggravates the other.

These people are most likely to have diseases of the heart and blood vessels, including high blood pressure; diabetes, overactive thyroid glands, and infections, primarily pneumonia.

There are four basic situations in which both types of illness occur concurrently:

- It may be just chance, and they are independent of each other
- There may be no known relationship, but they may be linked because of some irregularity in the body. Some researchers think, for example, that the same biochemical disturbance may contribute to both Parkinson's disease and depression.
- Other problems can be linked because they have

symptoms in common, such as anxiety and hyperthyroidism (an overactive thyroid gland)
- One problem may cause the other, like delirium as a result of serious physical illness

As one might suspect, depression is the most common psychiatric illness occurring simultaneously with physical illness. Thirty percent of the physically ill have emotional distress with sadness and anxiety, and between 15 and 20 percent develop a depressive illness. Yet it is often missed by the doctor treating the physical condition, because he or she figures the down mood, the loss of interest or pleasure in life, is a part of the normal grief and sadness that accompany illness, and will automatically go away with successful treatment of the physical condition.

However, if depression is treated as a separate entity, chances for recovery from it are very good.

Fifteen percent of the people who survive heart attacks are clinically depressed one year following their illness, 15 to 20 percent of those on artificial kidneys are depressed at any point in their treatment, 40 percent of cancer patients have depression. One-quarter of stroke patients have a major depression after their emergency, particularly if there has been damage to the left half of the brain; 30 percent have significant depression six months later, and some still have this mental problem two years after the stroke.

One theory to explain this is that some change in the structure or function of the nervous system, caused by the stroke, is the basis for the depression.

At least 20 percent of people with physical disorders also have alcohol or other drug-related problems, which understandably have complicating adverse effects on the nervous, digestive and cardiovascular systems.

Some attempts have been made to specify symptoms that are associated with depression, but are also expected as part of particular diseases. Loss of appetite and fatigue, for example, are common in cancer patients and are considered to be caused by the cancer. Loss of energy, insomnia and decreased sexual interest are common in kidney patients on dialysis, but loss of appetite and weight loss while the patient is on dialysis are considered indicative of a major depression.

Anxiety disorders, often linked with mild depressive symptoms, are the second most common condition occurring with physical disorders. Some diseases, such as hyperthyroidism, have common symptoms with anxiety. Delirium is thought to occur in 10 percent of patients hospitalized for medical conditions, and in 25 percent of elderly patients:

- they become disoriented
- their memory is impaired
- their sleep-wake cycle is altered
- they may have hallucinations

Delirium is often a sign of a serious physical illness, and about 25 percent of people die from the conditions which cause delirium. However, this illness can also be caused by medications themselves which were perhaps aimed at other problems.

The economic and social impact of concurrent psychiatric and physical disorders is substantial. These people make twice as many visits to doctors, their hospital stays are longer, they have five times as many referrals to specialists, and they are sent for more X-rays and lab tests. Their emotional illness may make them less likely to follow "doctor's orders" to improve their physical illness, and they are at higher risk for suicide. Depression may be a factor in their failure to return to work after a physical illness such as a heart attack, stroke, chronic kidney or obstructive lung disease.

There is also a significant emotional burden on the person, his family, and the doctors who are trying to sort out the patient's problems, and an additional dimension of financial stress can result when family members are unable to work because they are looking after the sick relative.

To provide a sense of the complexity involved here for doctors, Table 16.1 might be interesting. This information is taken from an article called "A Clinician's Guide to Differential Diagnosis Between Physical and Psychiatric Disorders," which was printed in the journal *Medical Psychotherapy* in 1988. The attempt here is to help the physician diagnose accurately.

Table 16.1 Survey of Major Elements of Interaction Between Physical and Mental Illnesses

Presenting Psychiatric Complaints or Symptoms	Suggested Psychiatric Diagnosis	If the Following Physical Sx are Present	Rule Out This Possible Physical Disorder	Recommended Lab Tests
Anxiety or Depression	Anxiety or Depression	Muscle spasms Increased tendon reflexes Tetany	Hypoparathyroidism	Serum calcium, phosphorus & magnesium levels 24-hour urinary calcium excretion Chest or bone X-rays Renal dye study
Anxiety or Depression	Anxiety or Depression	Somnolence Irritability Muscular weakness Gastrointestinal complaints Anorexia Nausea Constipation Renal stones Increased urinary output Abdominal pain	Hyperparathyroidism	
Depression Negativism Apathy Suspicion	Depression	Weight loss Loss of appetite Nausea Abdominal pain Recurrent diarrhea Decrease in strength Salt craving Muscle cramps Low blood pressure Loss of sex characteristics in females Increase in skin pigment	Hypoadrenalism (Addison's Disease)	Serum pituitary and adrenal Hormone levels Amount of 24-hour urinary excretion of endogenous steroids Dexamethasone Suppressant Test Adrenocorticotropic hormone (ACTH) stimulating test

Somatic Delusions Psychotic Thinking	Psychosis	Fatigue Emotional lability Incongruent weight gain with central deposits of fat and very thin limbs Acne Impotence / amenorrhea Large purple lines on the abdomen Easy bruising Hypertension Fragile skin Increased pigmentation Poor wound healing Increased urinary output	Hyperadrenalism (Cushing's Syndrome)	
Depressed Affect Lethargy Loss of Energy Delusions Hallucinations Paranoid Symptoms	Depression Schizophrenia	Weight gain Hypersomnia Cold intolerance Muscle aching Dry skin Hair loss Change in facial appearance Constipation Decrease in sexual functioning	Hypothyroidism	Thyroid Suppression Tests Tests of Thyroid Stim. Hormone Thyrotropin-Releasing Hormone Test Radioactive Iodine Uptake Test Measure levels of thyroxine, Tri-Iodothyromine, & level of blood serum protein
Episodic Anxiety Depression	Anxiety State Depression	Heat intolerance with excessive sweating Palpitations Tachycardia Fine rapid muscular tremor Weight loss Increased appetite combined with fatigue and weakness Bowel complaints Decreased menstrual flow Peculiar staring and prominence of patient's eyes	Hyperthyroidism	

Table 16.1 Survey of Major Elements of Interaction Between Physical and Mental Illnesses (continued)

Presenting Psychiatric Complaints or Symptoms	Suggested Psychiatric Diagnosis	If the Following Physical Sx are Present	Rule Out This Possible Physical Disorder	Recommended Lab Tests
Depression Lethargy Lack of energy Sense of weakness Inability to complete tasks	Depression	Bad breath Urine odor Eccentric food cravings	Diabetes mellitus	Fasting blood glucose levels Blood sugar challenge Glucose tolerance test
Fear Confusion Anxiety	Hysteria Dementia Anxiety Disorder Drug Intoxication	Tremulousness Sweating Heart palpitations Faintness Weakness	Excessive insulin levels	
Distractible Less careful about environment and personal hygiene	Personality Change Depression	Fatigue Weight loss Social withdrawal Insidious personality change Loss of recent memory Impaired immediate recall Inconsistent errors in calculating	Early Dementia (Chronic OBS)	Careful MSE with cognitive functioning evaluation Screening for Metabolic Abnormalities and Toxins EEG Lumbar Puncture and Lab Analysis of Cerebral Spinal Fluid CT Scan
Disorientation Auditory Hallucinations Visual Hallucinations Gait Problems	Psychosis Mania Schizophrenia	Causes: Stroke Severe Hypertension Wernicke-Korsakoff Syndrome Meningitis Encephalitis Severe hyperthyroidism Acute Adrenal Failure Poisoning	Delirium (Acute Confusional state or acute OBS)	

		ESP. Anticholinergics Hypoglycemia Vitamin deficiencies Systemic infections Renal failure Liver failure Blood electrolyte imbalance Subdural hematoma		
Confusion Disorientation Acting Out	Psychosis Delirium Explosive Personality Disorder Drug Reaction	Automatic behavior Lip smacking Clothes picking Wandering about Unaware of environment Violent outbursts Visual, olfactory, or auditory hallucinations	Seizure Disorder (Psychomotor or other temporal lobe)	EEG History and a therapeutic trial with anticonvulsant medication
Personality Change Depression Vague Neurologic or Endocrine Complaints	Dementia Depression	Gradual and Progressive Development of Sx including: Loss of social comp. Complaints of a new type of headache Specific loss of neurol. or muscle control Development of seizures during adulthood	Brain Tumor	CAT Scan Neurological Consult
Personality Change Increased Lethargy	Depression	Recent head trauma Hx of blackouts Decreased energy Decreasing activity levels (especially in elderly and alcoholics)	Subdural Hematoma	CAT Scan
Listlessness Irritability Periods of muscle weakness	Depression	Decreased muscle strength Easily fatigued	Myasthenia Gravis	Tensilon Test Electromyography or Serological Testing

Table 16.1 Survey of Major Elements of Interaction Between Physical and Mental Illnesses (continued)

Presenting Psychiatric Complaints or Symptoms	Suggested Psychiatric Diagnosis	If the Following Physical Sx are Present	Rule Out This Possible Physical Disorder	Recommended Lab Tests
Vague complaints of neurological losses	Hysteria/conversion Reaction	Repeated episodes in which the migratory nature of Sx becomes apparent and neurological losses become more persistent	Multiple Sclerosis	Exam of cerebral spinal fluid for protein and electrophoresis of the fluid
Complaint of numbness or pain with vague distribution Tiredness of a variable degree	Hypochondriasis	Complaints continue over time with only subtle changes in physical findings (Especially in alcoholics and Vitamin B deficiencies)	Peripheral Neuropathy	Nerve conduction studies Medical work-up
Dysphoric mood	Depression	Anorexia Weakness Fatigue Irritability Diffuse pain Unsteady walking gait Incoordination	Pernicious Anemia	Physical exam Blood count Shilling Test
Emotional Lability Sudden onsets of anxiety	Conversion Reaction Anxiety State	Colicky abdominal pain Vomiting Generalized weakness Seizures Rapid heart rate	Acute Porphyria	Blood test Barbiturate use Family history
Turmoil Adjustment Reactions Schizophrenic-like episodes	Anxiety Reaction Depression Psychosis	History of liver, renal or neurological disease Aggressive acting-out Mood swings Intellectual impairment	Wilson's Disease	Look for Kayser-Fleischer ring in cornea Levels of serum ceruloplasmin and copper
Depression	Depression	Unexplained physical complaints & findings	Tumor in a variety of organ systems	Physical evaluation

Depression	Depression	Development of liver complaints or Jaundice Dull, aching upper abdominal pain Constipation	Pancreatic Carcinoma	CAT Scan
Episodic Attacks Extreme Anxiety	Anxiety disorder	Hypertension Panic attacks Anxiety Perspiration Headache Tremor All without signs of neurotic adaptations	Pheochromocytoma (Adrenal Tumor) or Carcinoid Tumor	24-hour collections of urine for specific metabolites
Hallucinations Delusions Agitation Difficulty in associations Flight of ideas Vague symptoms of somatic origin	Schizophrenia Hysteria/Conversion Disorder	Labile rather than flat affect Unexplained fever Skin rash Arthritis Chest and abdominal complaints	Systemic Lupus Erythematous	Serologic tests Skin and tissue biopsies
Agitation	Mania	Fever Other complications compatible with viral infection	Viral Infections (influenza, Q fever, post-St. Louis type A Encephalitis)	Blood tests dependent on site & type of infection
Depression	Depression	Fever Masses Symptoms of localized infection	Bacterial Infection	

* * * Treatment

Techniques aimed at coping directly with the physical disorder, to limit its severity and the manifestations of its symptoms, have shown promise of also reducing anxiety or depression in people with diseases like high blood pressure, coronary heart disease, asthma, peptic ulcers, ulcerative colitis and irritable bowel syndrome. These approaches can include education about the illness, relaxation training, psychological support and behavioral therapy.

Group support programs for those with heart attacks, diabetes, kidney disease, cancer, and chronic obstructive lung disease have indicated an improved adjustment to the illness, but have not proven effective in preventing psychiatric disorders from developing. The usual treatment for depression, in those who are not also physically ill, has a 70 percent improvement rate, but this drops to only about 40 percent when concurrent illnesses are present.

Such diminished effectiveness can be due to medical complications, the impact of drugs being given for the physical illness, or the rapid appearance of side effects from anti-depressants, so they cannot be given in adequate doses.

In cases of major depression, when drugs are not tolerated, electroconvulsive therapy may be an alternative. Anxiety disorders can be alleviated with treatment of the medical condition that preceded them, such as an overactive thyroid gland, or some types of seizures, as well as the usual treatments for anxiety, panic and phobic disorders in people who have no other physical illness.

In delirium, treatment includes dealing with the medical problem, improving sleeping patterns, and an anti-psychotic drug. Children with medical disabilities, such as a physical deformity or epilepsy, should be brought up as normally as possible so that they can develop an identity as "a person with epilepsy" rather than an "epileptic."

At the same time they may need special support to participate in regular activities. For example, a child with epilepsy should be taught never to swim alone; one with diabetes should be instructed to always have food or drink on hand to correct a sudden insulin reaction.

*** Research

Scientific study in this area has been hampered by the complexities of the interactions between physical and psychological disorders, and the great diversity among patients. It is difficult to find enough people in exactly the same situation in order to do studies that are statistically meaningful.

The first step would be to perform studies to define the extent of the problem, combined with long-term follow-up to monitor the outcome of any treatments the patients receive.

The power of intervention could then be studied by giving one group of caregivers an educational package about a particular psychiatric or medical disorder, and comparing that group to another without this information, in terms of the success of treatment practices.

Unfortunately, far more research is needed on the effects of psychoactive drugs on the elderly and the physically ill. It is usually young and healthy volunteers who are used to test the safety and efficacy of such products.

Chapter 17

Suicide

Suicide is the ultimate expression of despair.

We inwardly recoil when we hear that someone has killed himself, not wanting to accept that someone can be so bereft of hope that he is unwilling to face any possible tomorrow.

Yet the numbers are troubling. For example, in Canada the annual death rate from suicide, at 15 per 100,000 population, is higher than that from diabetes, cirrhosis of the liver, or kidney disease. In Canada alone suicide accounts for more than 3,000 deaths a year.

In the US, with a population ten times larger, the annual figure turns out to also be roughly ten fold greater: approximately 30,000 annually. And these are just the deaths recognized as suicides: some current studies show the actual rate is underestimated by at least 20 percent. Sometimes they are disguised as accidents. Coroners certifying a cause of death may yield to pressures to render this verdict where there is any doubt whatsoever, in order to spare the family of the victim additional pain.

Perhaps even more distressing than the loss of lives is the loss of potential years of life for these individuals and the country, because suicide has been increasing among young people. An interesting study quantified this situation in Canada, to provide some sense of the social costs involved. When the age at suicide was compared with the normal life span of 70 years, two million life-years were lost to Canadians between 1963 and 1976. This tragic event robs females of more years of potential life than any other cause, and in men is second only to heart attacks.

Suicide rates vary widely throughout the world. Canada's 15 per 100,000 recently overtook the American rate of 13 per 100,000. Hungary's is in the 40s, and Greece is at the bottom of the list with three. The Scandinavian countries, except Norway, range from 20s to 30s, and predominantly Catholic countries like Ireland, Italy and Mexico have low suicide rates.

*** *Causes*

As would be suspected from the divergent suicide rates in different countries, cultural and environmental factors can play a role in one's vulnerability to suicide, but there are also important psychological and biological factors to be considered.

To a small degree, suicides tend to run in families. If one identical twin takes his or her own life, in 18 cases of 100 so will the other. A Danish-American study of children adopted in infancy showed those who committed suicide were more likely to have a blood relative who had killed himself, indicating a genetic factor.

Although it seems unlikely that there would be a specific genetic factor for suicide, independent of depression or other mental disorders, there does seem to be a separate genetic component. Suicide in the absence of a severe disorder is rare, but given a person with a psychiatric disorder, the likelihood of suicide is greater if a family member has killed himself in the past. The nature of this genetic tendency is not presently known, but some people think it may involve impulsiveness. A person with this characteristic, who is also depressed, is more likely to act on a suicidal urge than one who has greater self-control. It is plausible that impulsiveness might be inherited.

Alcoholics have a suicide rate which is an incredible 80 times higher than the norm. Many start drinking as a home remedy for depression, and then drinking becomes an end in itself. Their choice of alcohol as a treatment is a poor one, since it is itself a depressant, and chronic alcoholism is known to induce depression, probably contributing to this high suicide rate. In addition, alcoholics often commit what could be called accidental suicide, by taking an overdose of sleeping pills or other medications while their judgment and perception are impaired by intoxication.

People who have personality disorders, or who misuse illicit drugs, are 20 times more likely than the norm to commit suicide. Often only after they kill themselves is it recognized that they had severe problems maintaining relationships because of the difficulties they experienced with their own personalities.

Numerous "psychological autopsies" of suicides, done by interviews with families and friends after death, indicate that in the vast majority of cases some mental illness was involved. Most often this was depressive illness, but alcoholism, schizophrenia and organic brain disease were also well represented. A fatal medical illness was a factor in only five percent of these cases, and in a mere four percent was no mental illness at all discovered. Depressed people have an overwhelming sense of pessimism, hopelessness and helplessness, which can be relieved with treatment, but since they usually do not realize that their feelings stem from their illness, they often do not seek medical or psychiatric help.

As suggested by research summarized in Figure 17.1, depression is a major factor in suicides.

Figure 17.1
Diagnoses in 440 Patients Who Had Attempted Suicide

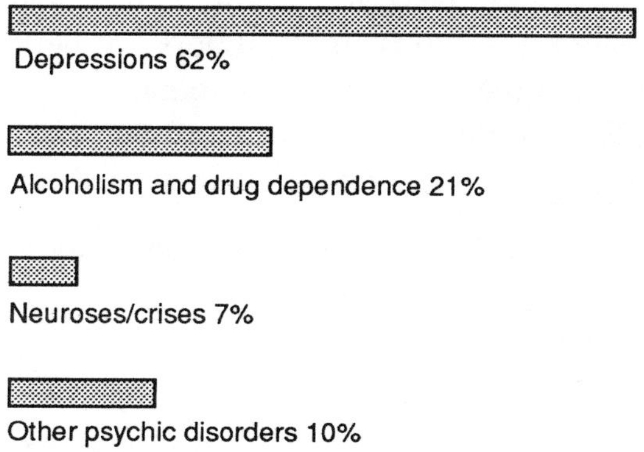

Source: Pöldinger, W.J. (1989). The Psychopathology and Psychodynamics of Self-Destruction. *Crisis,* 10: 113-122.

A 19th-century sociologist, Emile Durkheim, observed that united and cohesive societies, with high morale and collective ideals, have low suicide rates. Rates are high in those societies torn apart by chaos, where values are obscured, standards of conduct are in disarray, and the result is what he termed "anomie." People do not feel that they have an accepted place in their own community, and the result is "every man for himself."

Sometimes the value system of a particular society can become so distorted as to even decree suicide, as in the mass suicide tragedy of the followers of the Rev. Jim Jones in Guyana.

Interestingly, suicide rates fell during the two world wars, probably because people had a greater feeling of pulling together in a common cause. But during these years there was also fuller employment, another major factor that affects suicide rates.

Care must be taken to avoid automatically labelling statistical relationships as causes, for example, as with the positive association between unemployment and suicide. Obviously not everyone who falls into a certain category commits suicide, but viable patterns do emerge.

Recent Canadian studies which compared suicide rates across various provinces at one point in time, and at a 10-year interval, showed suicide was clearly linked to divorce, alcoholism, social isolation, and lack of integration. The provinces with the greatest increases in suicide over the decade also had higher unemployment, but, at the same time, greater affluence on average in the population. It would seem that people are more vulnerable to suicide when their neighbors are better off, than when everyone is in the same economic boat.

A Canadian government-appointed task force, asked to identify high-risk groups, defined them in a 1987 report as:

- those with a mental disorder (including alcoholism)
- young people
- the elderly
- native peoples
- those in prison

Throughout North America there is a startling increase in suicide among teenagers and young adults, who also have increased rates of depression and related illnesses, including drug abuse and alcoholism. Males aged 15 to 24 are at the highest risk among the young group, but suicides by those aged 5 to 14 are also on the rise. These youngsters usually choose some violent means of ending their lives.

The elderly account for 10 percent of all suicides. Factors including Alzheimer's Disease, depression, failing health, loneliness, idleness, and inadequate income may all lead to a feeling of hopelessness.

An incredible thirty-six percent of the deaths among native people are violent ones, many of them suicides. Sixty percent of young native people 15 to 24 who die do so at their own hands, half

Table 17.1
Data on Suicide for Native versus All Canadians Populations

	Natives	All Canadians
Death rate per 100,000 — 1987	965	650
Infant death rate (under one year) per 1,000 — 1986	17.4	7.9
Death by injury and poisoning (including drunk driving fatalities) per 100,000 — 1987	216	54.4
Death by suicide per 100,000	1984-'88	1984-'87
All ages	36.1	13.8
15 - 19	65.7	12.3
20 - 24	94.3	18.3
25 - 29	64.4	18.3
Death by respiratory diseases (caused partly by poor housing) per 100,000 — 1987	90.5	49.8
Death by infectious and parasitic diseases (including TB, caused by poor diet, poor sanitation, etc.) per 100,000	15.6	4.3
Average life expectancy at birth — 1984-'86	65.9 yrs.	75 yrs.

Source: Canada Health and Welfare Department, Statistics Canada, Assembly of First Nations of them by shooting themselves. Other comparisons are shown in Table 17.1. For example, natives aged 15-19 are more than five times as likely to take their own lives versus Canadians in general.

Aside from these groupings, the statistically most likely person to commit suicide is a divorced, unemployed man of any race or nationality, over 45, living alone, and recently discharged from a hospital.

Unfortunately, one must ultimately accept that many suicides are not preventable, even when the victim had received a high degree of affection, care and attention from family, friends and members of the medical profession. More might be prevented if their despair was recognized earlier as part of a treatable psychiatric disorder.

*** *Attempted Suicide*

Attempted suicide, "parasuicide" as mental health professionals call it, is usually not a determined try, but it should never be taken lightly, because a more serious, and successful, attempt could follow.

Eight times as many people make suicide attempts as those who manage to kill themselves, and most parasuicides are young females. In contrast, as one ages the likelihood of actually achieving death rises, as suggested by research summarized in Figure 17.2.

Many people take drug overdoses or cut their wrists as a call for help in resolving their problems, taking precautions so they will be discovered in time. But unfortunately a large number of these people will indeed kill themselves eventually if their lives do not improve.

Those who deliberately try to hurt themselves report four times as many stressful life events in the preceding six months as normal people. They generally have poor coping skills, and their personal lives are often very disorganized. They are likely to have a background of child abuse, childhood losses, and to have witnessed the effects of self-harm in other people they knew. From a recent book on this subject, a number of clear behavioral

Figure 17.2
Age Distribution of Patients Committing Suicide (—) or Attempting Suicide (—)

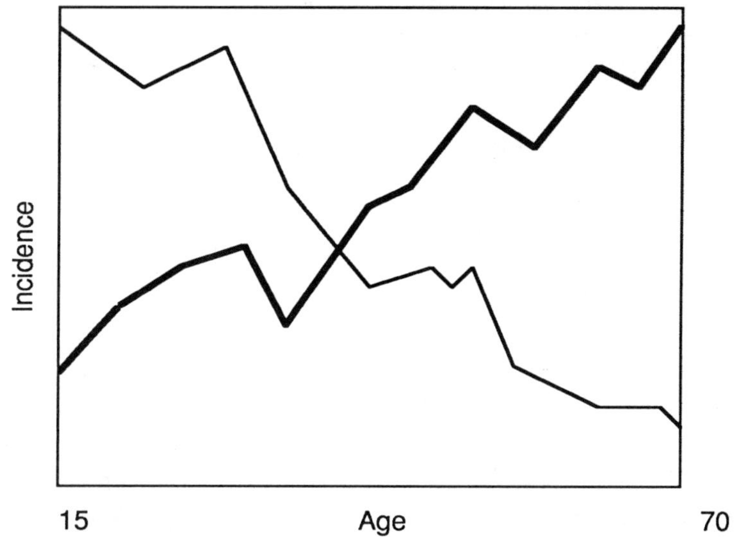

Source: Pöldinger, W.J. (1989). The Psychopathology and Psychodynamics of Self-Destruction. *Crisis,* 10: 113-122.

and communication indicators of serious intent to commit suicide have been determined:

Behavioral Indicators:

- Loss of interest in former activities; withdrawal from social contact
- Difficulty in concentrating
- Problems with judgment and memory
- A dramatic shift in the quality of schoolwork and academic performance
- Feelings of sadness, emptiness and hopelessness, which may be expressed in the student's written assignments
- Sleep disturbances, frequently insomnia but also hypersomnia

- Overt expression of anger and rage, ranging from intense verbal outbursts to physical aggression
- Excessive use of drugs and/or alcohol
- Promiscuous behavior
- Uncharacteristic delinquent behavior; thrill-seeking
- Absence of known deterrents, such as friends and family

Verbal or non-verbal communication indicators may include:

- Occurrence of previous suicidal gestures or attempts
- Statements revealing a desire to die or a preoccupation with death (may also be obvious in written assignments)
- Nihilistic comments; life is meaningless, filled with misery
- Verbal or written threats
- Gestures to be noticed (self-mutilation, scratches)
- Planning for death, making final arrangements, giving away favorite personal possessions
- Suddenly becoming cheerful after prolonged depression may represent "relief" that the decision is taken

*** Prevention

Factors that encourage suicide, like unemployment, are not easy to remedy, but governments can reduce the hardship and humiliation that can accompany these social problems. It is also possible for governments to restrict access to some of the more lethal methods of suicide, which can be used impulsively. One-third of North American suicides result from gunshot wounds, and as one might suspect, lower suicide rates have followed tighter gun control in some U.S. states.

Sticking one's head in the gas oven was a common method of suicide in the United Kingdom until the 1960s, when the country switched to supplies of non-toxic natural gas. People still continued to attempt suicide in this manner, and as a result, the successful suicide rate fell dramatically. In addition, suicides using carbon monoxide from car exhaust were highest from the 1950s through the 1960s, then declined when cars were equipped with catalytic converters and other emission control devices. Use of this method began to rise again when people were able to determine how to disconnect these devices from their automobiles. The number of suicides from the Golden Gate Bridge in San Francisco was reduced when access to a jumping-off point was made more difficult. The establishment of a system to make it difficult to jump in front of an oncoming subway train might have similar results.

Less media attention to suicides might also help, since people in very disturbed states tend to imitate suicides. Improved access to help for the emotionally disturbed, including assessment, treatment and follow-up care, as well as education to deflate the stigma of mental illness, could also help cut the death toll.

In addition, and very importantly, communities could take very specific steps to develop programs which lessen the isolation of the young, the old, and native people so they no longer feel friendless. Indeed this may be one of the most productive areas which can receive further attention.

There is no doubt that some form of intervention is needed when people are expressing suicidal intentions, or have already harmed themselves. Psychiatrists are not always required at this stage, because other physicians, nurses and social workers can be effective if they are adequately trained. Properly trained volunteers manning telephone help lines can also screen and refer suicidal people for care. A new book by experts in this area presents specific techniques which can be used by a wide variety of physicians, allied health professionals and lay people involved with suicide prevention [see MacLean in the references]. But the incidence of the problem, and the social costs involved are so high that developing a far greater range of effective methods would be highly productive.

Specialized psychiatric units in general hospitals which provide intensive assessment and short-term treatments can deal not only with crisis situations, but can also provide valuable training for staff and students, as well as community members.

In considering the many aspects of this problem, some larger cities have formed groups for those who are left behind after a successful suicide. These are staffed by bereavement counselors, to help those who have been left in an emotional catastrophe by the suicide of a friend or relative. They can share their anger, sadness, bafflement, and sense of overwhelming guilt with others who have gone through this experience, and dealt with the inevitable feeling of blame: "If only I had...." Such suffering is especially great for parents who lose a child to suicide. Many feel that the burden of this experience is the worst imaginable suffering, which virtually never subsides, even years after the event.

*** Research

Overall, the incidence of this problem is so great, and the social costs so severe, that far more effort to solve the problem would undoubtedly be highly productive.

Much greater understanding of all the disorders linked to suicide is needed [see the chapters on Addictions, Depression and Schizophrenia], as well as further studies on how specific risk factors are determined.

A decade ago, in a series of interesting studies, Swedish researchers found that depressed patients who attempted suicide had remarkably lower levels of the breakdown product or metabolite of serotonin, one of the chemical messengers in the central nervous system. Far more research is needed into the possibility that suicide may be associated with low serotonin in the brain. The same shortage has since been found in people who have attempted suicides, who are also suffering from other mental illnesses, such as schizophrenia and personality disorders. Anomalies in serotonin have been found in post-mortem brain examination of suicides.

Serotonin is also believed to play a large role in regulating mood, aggression, sexual behavior, appetite and sleep. It has been found that low levels of the metabolite are associated with violent crimes committed on sudden impulse, and these same low levels are more often found among those who try suicide impulsively and by violent methods. This leads to speculation that a malfunction in the serotonin system can cause sudden loss of control over aggression, which can be unleashed against oneself or others. Alcohol is also known to affect serotonin levels in the brain. More study of the chemistry and regulation of this substance might lead to development of medications which would elevate it to normal levels, and help keep it there.

While there have been a variety of new social policies targeted to reduce the isolation of groups which are vulnerable to suicide, these have not yet been adequately evaluated for their effect on the suicide rate.

*** For Further Information

American Association of Suicidology, 2459 S. Ash., Denver, Colorado 80222

Canadian Association of Suicide Prevention, P.O. Box 56, Station 'K', Toronto, Ontario M4P 2G1

The Council on Suicide Prevention, 10 Trinity Square, Toronto, Ontario, M5G 1B1.

A Handbook for the Caregiver on Suicide Prevention, by the Council of Suicide Prevention, Hamilton and District. Available through the Board of Education, City of Hamilton, P.O. Box 558, 100 Main Street West, Hamilton, Ontario L8L 3L1.

Hawton, K.H., and Catalan, J. (1987). *Attempted Suicide*. New York: Oxford University Press.

MacLean, Dr. George A., editor. (1990). *Suicide in Children and Adolescents*. Toronto: Hogrefe& Huber Publishers.

Suicide in Canada: A Report of the National Task Force. (1987). Health and Welfare Canada.

Chapter 18

Psychiatry and the Law

At 2:00 am, two men are in a hospital emergency department. One has come because he is so depressed that he sees no point in living — he considers himself worthless. The other is having severe chest pains, and examination shows he has just had a heart attack. Both men are told they should be admitted, and both refuse.

The man with the heart attack will be allowed to leave, probably after signing a statement to the effect that he is doing so against medical advice. The man with the depression might very well be hospitalized against his will under local laws which provide for the involuntary treatment of anyone considered to have a mental disorder and to be a danger to himself or others.

Yet either man, if he drives away from the hospital, may put himself and others in jeopardy. The depressed one could drive his car into another in a suicide attempt; the heart attack victim could lose control of his car and go careening into oncoming traffic.

This scenario illustrates that society still makes major distinctions between physical and mental illnesses, and their treatments, based on the assumption that only a mental disorder interferes with the ability to give informed consent to treatment. Those distinctions also put psychiatrists into roles which often bring them into conflict with each other, with other physicians, and with society.

When a mentally ill person is unable to make judgments about his or her own physical welfare, these decisions are usually made by the consensus of a group of physicians until the person is again capable of such decisions.

In North America it is generally believed that society has both a responsibility and a right to protect people from themselves and from others. This right can be exercised in a "parental" role, as happens under mental health legislation, when someone who needs care appears unable or unwilling to seek it for himself. In other cases, society can exercise a police power under the Criminal Code: those perceived as being mentally ill and dangerous can be legally compelled to have psychiatric assessment and treatment.

Unfortunately, it is often assumed that psychiatric patients are more dangerous than patients with other illnesses, even though studies show otherwise. One reason may be that we tend to fear people whose behavior can be unpredictable, or bizarre, or whose appearance may be different than what is considered "normal."

Another reason is probably the extensive media coverage given to cases when a psychiatric patient does commit a serious crime such as murder. Stereotypes about certain ethnic or social groups are reinforced when one member of them commits a crime, but, for example, most motorcyclists are not criminals, and most schizophrenics are withdrawn rather than aggressive.

Generally, a doctor's principal duty is to a patient's welfare, but in some circumstances he or she may be obliged to put society's needs first. In accordance with certain laws a doctor must report a patient who is medically unfit to pilot a plane or drive a car, or who has one of a designated group of communicable diseases, to the appropriate government authority.

Psychiatrists, on the other hand, are often called upon to give opinions regarding people who may or may not be their patients, in order to help those within the legal system to make decisions.

Legal Implications in Canada

Local mental health laws vary quite a bit, but in general, they provide for the involuntary admission of a person to a psychiatric unit if he or she has a mental disorder and is considered a danger to himself or others. This is usually called "being committed." Depending on the location in North America, medical doctors, and certain mental health professionals who are employed by the local government, have the power to decide if a person meets these conditions and should be admitted. In other locations only a physician who is also a psychiatrist has this legal power. In many, but not all situations, two opinions from separate examinations are needed to arrive at the decision to commit a patient for psychiatric assessment.

In many cases, as much force as is necessary can be used to take a person to a mental hospital without his consent. In some situations the person may also be treated without his consent, after a review of the case by a committee or a board.

These powers have always been debated. Free societies place a high value on personal liberty, yet they also have responsibilities to all of their citizens. Periodic revisions of mental health legislation usually attempt to improve the balance between these conflicting obligations, and are often criticized as having gone too far in the direction of leniency or of restrictiveness. Psychiatrists are often accused of being arbitrary restrictors of liberty in this role, yet they are compelled by law to make involuntary admissions in certain circumstances.

They also may be asked to give an opinion about whether or not an accused person is fit to stand trial — whether he or she can understand the charge and the court procedure, and is able to instruct a lawyer. If it is suspected that the person is not fit because of mental illness, a psychiatrist is asked to make an examination and give an opinion. On the basis of this information, it is the court which then decides if, in fact, the accused person is fit. If the court declares that the accused is not mentally capable, he is sent to a psychiatric facility for up to 60 days for further examination and possible treatment.

After that, he goes back to court with a report from the examining psychiatrist at the facility, and the court again decides if he is capable to stand trial. If not, in Canada he is returned to a psychiatric institution under a Lieutenant-Governor's warrant. Theoretically, that means he can be kept in the institution indefinitely, but the Criminal Code provides for boards that review all of these patients' situations at least once a year. These boards normally include a lawyer or judge, two psychiatrists and a lay member of the community. The patient is represented by a lawyer, and the board considers the opinions of the psychiatrist in charge of the patient, given under oath.

When the criminal trial actually takes place, a psychiatrist may be required to give an opinion as to whether the accused had the mental capacity to form the intent to commit the crime, or if he was in touch with reality when committing it. Could the crime have been the result of a serious mental illness, like a deluded person attacking a stranger whom he really believed was a bear about to devour him? It is up to the judge, or judge and jury, to decide whether a person can be held responsible for his crime. In Canada, a person cannot be held responsible for a crime when declared insane, but the definition of "insanity" in the Criminal Code is a legal one, not a medical one.

A person judged "not guilty by reason of insanity" is confined to a mental hospital under a Lieutenant-Governor's warrant.

During its periodic assessments over the course of a confinement, the review board recommends whether the person should be released, whether his confinement should be less restrictive, or whether he should continue to be fully confined.

This recommendation goes to the provincial justice department, which then makes its own recommendation to the provincial cabinet, which in turn technically makes its recommendation to the Lieutenant-Governor, who then makes the final decision about the release or continued confinement of the person. Needless to say all this is incredibly expensive, but it underscores the value which is placed on individual choice and responsibility, since if the person is regarded as being in control of his actions, he is held accountable. But because of these safeguards, cases still occur where horrible crimes can be committed and yet the offender is treated, rather than punished in the more usual sense.

Indeed, in criminal trials, psychiatrists are often called upon at the time of sentencing to give an opinion about the realistic treatment and rehabilitation alternatives, in order to assist the court in deciding on an appropriate disposition of the case.

In Canada psychiatric testimony is also required by law in applications under the Dangerous Offenders Act. If a court declares a person to be a dangerous offender it can sentence him to an indeterminate period in an institution. He will be confined forever unless a parole board decides otherwise. Sentences are normally reviewed after three years, and every two years thereafter.

To declare someone a dangerous offender, it must be shown that he is indeed dangerous — that he would probably commit similar offenses again, and that his conduct is harmful to others. Two psychiatrists, one for the defense and one for the Crown, must testify as to whether he meets these two conditions.

In both the US and Canada this type of situation can place psychiatrists in difficult ethical dilemmas because they are required by law to predict the future behavior of individuals, and possible harm to potential victims, and there is as yet no scientific knowledge on which such predictions can be based.

It is easy to describe dangerous behavior. A person running amok in the street angrily swinging a meat cleaver is behaving dangerously. But to predict dangerous conduct — to say that a certain person might well run amok with a meat cleaver at some time in the future — is a totally different matter.

Legal Implications in the United States

In the US the procedural steps are quite like those in Canada, because law in both countries evolved from the English common law system. But there are differences, which in turn vary quite a bit among individual regions.

In most states the insanity defense is the same, as it is derived from English law, although in 1954 Judge David Bazelon of the District of Columbia Court of Appeals wrote the famous Durham decision which says simply that an accused is not criminally responsible if his unlawful act is the product of mental disease or defect. In 1984 Congress enacted the Insanity Defense Reform Act which brought uniformity to the variety of different regulations in different states. It refines the Durham decision by stating that if the defendant at the time of the commission of the act constituting the offence suffered from a severe mental disease or defect and was therefore unable to appreciate the nature and quality or wrongfulness of his acts, then he is not legally responsible. Upon such a conviction such patients are ordinarily transferred to the custody of their own state hospital system where they can then be involuntarily hospitalized in accordance with civil commitment proceedings. In many states, such a commitment can be only for a short period.

In some states (Alaska, Connecticut, Georgia, Illinois, Indiana, Kentucky, Michigan and New Mexico) a new verdict of "guilty but mentally ill" has been adopted, while still retaining a verdict of not guilty by reason of insanity. The implication is that the convicted will receive treatment for mental illness, but this is not mandatory. Both the American Psychiatric Association in 1982, and the American Bar Association in 1986, expressed their opposition to the addition of "guilty but mentally ill."

Competency to Stand Trial. Most state laws specify that the incompetency must be the result of mental disease or defect. If found incompetent the defendant is usually committed to a mental institution for treatment. When competency is restored he may then go to trial and be found guilty, unless it was determined that he was insane at the time of the offence. However, the period of confinement is limited, and institutions are forced to restore competency by adequate treatment and return the defendant for trial at the earliest possible time.

Involuntary Hospitalization. In recent decades, safeguards to the misuse of involuntary commitment of hospitalization have been introduced. While previous commitment periods were measured in months and years, new procedures speak only of hours and days of involuntary confinement. After an initial 72 hour period of observation, patients could be involuntarily detained for two weeks if found dangerous to themselves or others, or to be gravely disabled. This decision is made by the staff of the mental health facility. A patient who is actively suicidal could be detained for another two week period. No commitment provisions were made for longer term hospitalization for disabled patients, but instead a concept of conservatorship was developed. A conservator has less power than a guardian and acquires only limited powers. The conservator has the authority to have the conservatee admitted to a hospital as a voluntary patient and to act as a substitute decision maker in consenting for treatment. The period of conservatorship is limited by statute — in California, it is one year, and only allowed for a grave disability, which is defined as the inability because of mental disease to provide food, clothing and shelter for one's self.

Some states have additional commitment procedures for sexual psychopaths or disordered sex offenders. The national trend is away from such specialized commitments, but there are now new commitment procedures for mentally disordered violent offenders which permit the confinement of such people to continue after their prison terms have expired. All states and the District of Columbia have provisions for the commitment of offenders determined to be incompetent to stand trial or not guilty by reason of insanity. There is a new type of involuntary commitment for outpatients which requires a patient to attend the clinic as often as needed for therapy or regulation of medication, but does not otherwise restrict their activities.

Right to Treatment. In 1960, it was suggested that involuntarily institutionalized patients have a constitutional right to treatment, and this could provide a means of forcing states to meet at least minimum standards for care and treatment. This was first established in a Federal Court in 1972.

Overall, this broad area where psychiatry and the law interact is an ambiguous one. Like other kinds of physicians, psychiatrists have scientific knowledge and expertise to recognize and treat illness, but they are often quite uncomfortable with the role of social agent, which is often imposed on them by legal statutes. This is especially true in psychiatry, a science which has made tremendous gains in the last 30 years, but certainly still has difficulty in perfectly predicting human behavior.

*** Research

The sort of breakthroughs required in this area are not the kind which are done in a laboratory. What is needed is a far greater understanding of how to achieve much better communications, to narrow the gulf between the legal and medical systems, and to develop problem-solving techniques that best serve both public protection and individual rights.

Institutes of law and medicine are grappling with these problems, and a new field is developing which lies somewhere between the two, concerning itself with the ethics of legal practice and health policy. Experts in this new field have plenty of material to examine, even if current legal issues are eventually resolved. In addition, as genetic molecular biology plays an expanding role in psychiatric research, society will be faced with more questions of the kind: "Although we now can do it, should we do it?" For example:

- If it is found that fetal brain tissue transplants can cure some brain deficiencies, should aborted fetuses be used for this purpose?

- If a test becomes available that would show a pregnant woman that her child has a substantial chance of developing schizophrenia, to whom should the test be offered, and how should pregnant women be counseled?

- Will the constant search for cost containment and cost-effectiveness result in criticism of or sanctions against women who either refuse to take these tests, or to act "appropriately" on the results?

Legal scholars are grappling with another thorny issue — what criteria should be used as a basis for involuntary commitment to a hospital for a person with a psychiatric disorder? Most jurisdictions rely on a judgment that the person is a danger to him or herself or to others. Most people with psychiatric disorders are not dangerous, but many lose insight during their illness and do not realize that they are ill. Thus, they fail to seek help and suffer greatly.

Some legal practitioners argue that the present laws deprive patients of an important right — the right to treatment. The difficult task for legal scholars is to define "loss of insight," which is a medical condition, as a form of legal incompetence. In other words, when a person becomes incompetent to act in the interest of his or her own health, can a legal definition be made, accurately describing this state, which does not also jeopardize the fundamental rights of healthy people?

Chapter 19

Getting Help

The case studies in this book show that it is often difficult to tell at the beginning of a psychiatric disorder that a major problem is actually developing. It is quite normal to be sad or anxious or confused at times, for example, but just how long should one wait before seeking help?

Initially, family and good friends try their best. But when the person can clearly not be cheered up or calmed down, and the problem goes on and on, they start to feel helpless, frustrated and even impatient. They come to wish that the problem would go away, or the person would seek help somewhere else. This is a perfectly natural reaction, and it's also a signal that professional assistance may be needed.

But often people do not realize that they need help. They have already made up their minds about the problem... if only someone else would change, if only they were under less stress, if only a certain unfortunate event had not happened in the past, and so on...

At this stage, many people become willing to turn to the first line of defense in the care system, one of the self-help groups that fortunately abound in most communities. Some of them are listed at the end of appropriate chapters in this book. The Canadian and American Mental Health Associations, listed in the white pages of most telephone books, can make suggestions about those which are locally available.

In addition, members of the clergy are often well trained in mental health issues, and they may be able to help a person through a crisis, or provide excellent direction to other sources of help if the problem is more serious.

Another alternative is the relatively new employee assistance programs or EAPs, which are being made increasingly available in the workplace. Originally designed to help employees with alcohol or other substance abuse problems, they have evolved to cover a wide range of circumstances. Businesses hire counselors — often psychologists or social workers — with whom an employee or family member can confidentially discuss difficulties, because these consultants do not report back to the employer. The counselors may be able to help with the problem themselves, or refer the person to an appropriate community resource.

Family doctors are also in a good position to spot problems, because they have often known patients and their families for years. They are well acquainted with the way people react to changes in the life cycle, like adolescence, getting married and retiring, and they are familiar with how people react to hazardous events like accidents or death. They are often capable of providing short-term psychotherapy to help a person through such crises. Individual family doctors do vary in the training and interest they have in this field, so some will get more involved than others, but they can advise a patient when he or she should see a psychiatrist, and a patient may be more willing to accept such a suggestion when it comes from a doctor they know and trust.

Figure 19.1 below illustrates the broad variety of facilities available to help deal with the mentally ill, from the highly specialized state or provincial psychiatric hospital, to nursing homes and primary care physicians. The intensity of use of these arrangements is suggested by the schematic line, showing that few people end up using the police, while a much larger number become involved with primary care providers.

Some family physicians work with psychologists who help them deal with the common emotional problems of everyday life, and help them assess more serious difficulties. When problems become extreme, help is required urgently and quickly. The American Psychiatric Association has recently published 10 warning signs of mental illness, signs that things have gone

Figure 19.1
Intensity of Use of Civilian Institutions Dealing with Mental Health

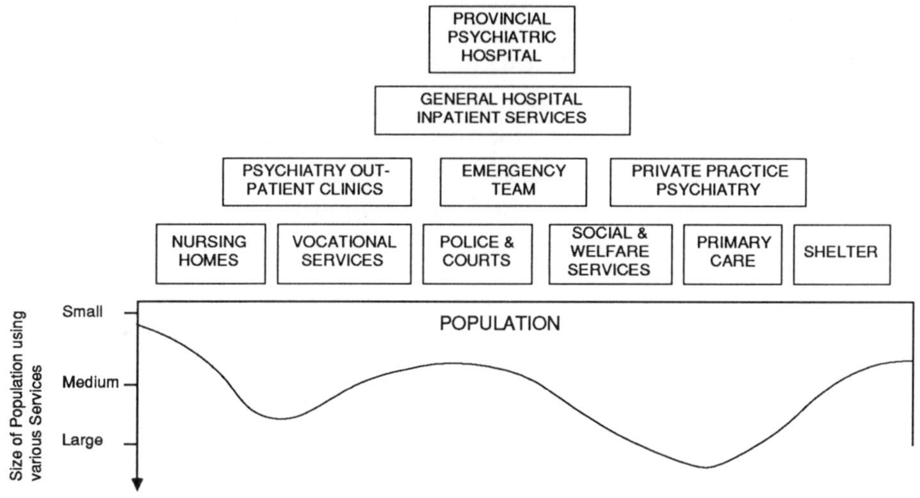

beyond an ordinary life crisis. These warning signs are:

- marked and persistent personality change
- persistent inability to cope with problems in daily activities
- persistent strange and grandiose ideas
- persistent and excessive anxiety
- prolonged depression and apathy
- marked changes in sleeping or eating patterns
- thinking or talking about suicide
- extreme highs or lows of mood
- abuse of alcohol or other drugs
- excessive hostility, anger or violent behavior

Any one of these situations warrants assessment and treatment, and a referral to a psychiatrist or a psychiatric outpatient clinic. If the situation is urgent, a hospital emergency room is the best place to go, since the people there will be able to treat most immediate physical problems, and then find additional sources of help.

Contrary to popular belief, most psychiatrically troubled people are not very dangerous to others, and therefore relatively few individuals enter psychiatric care through the legal system, as did the patient with mania described in the chapter on depression. Because he was totally unaware that he had a problem, it was only when he became abusive toward an officer after being stopped for a traffic violation that he was provided with the psychiatric care he needed.

*** Getting Healthier

Mental health is more than the absence of mental illness and non-medical mental health workers often feel psychiatrists don't place enough emphasis on mental health. They believe it is the responsibility of individuals, the groups to which they belong, and the larger social environment, to interact in a way that makes people feel well and use their human potential to the fullest. This includes not only their intelligence, but also their emotional capabilities, and the ability to have satisfying and constructive relationships.

Innumerable case studies have shown that individuals can indeed acquire new skills and resources to enable them to meet their personal needs, and to also contribute to society. This is true not only of people who are healthy in the first place, but also of those who have experienced a mental illness.

Many individuals who have recovered can continue to grow beyond the degree of health they had before the illness started. Even if theirs is a recurrent condition, the rest of their lives need not continue to be scarred by the history of past illness, and they can be exceptionally healthy in the periods between recurrences.

Conversely, a person may have clinically recovered from a

severe mental problem, but still not have returned to good mental health. Perhaps his friends and family have rejected him. He may feel stigmatized by his illness and be unable to find or keep suitable housing or employment. He may also lack social, recreational and educational opportunities, coping skills, and the vital information he needs to correct these circumstances.

Poverty is a classic example of a social condition that contributes to mental health problems, whether or not one has previously had a mental illness. Inadequate housing is another.

Institutionalization is no longer the nightmare it was at the turn of the century. Mental hospitals today are smaller and better staffed than in the past, due in large part to the development of effective medications in the 1950s. But a different problem has developed, particularly in large cities, where patients who were formerly in institutions now live in ghettos of boarding houses or literally on the streets, completely neglected by their families and by society. Thousands live in squalor and poverty, with few defenses against exploitation.

This situation is worsened by the tightening of laws that prohibit the hospitalization of patients against their will, except for a brief assessment period for those who may be dangerous to themselves or others. Indeed, quite a bit of tension has been developing in North America, between those whose primary concerns are the protection of individual rights, and those mental health professionals, and often family members, who know someone is ill but are aware that the person lacks enough insight into that illness to agree to seek care.

As with all sicknesses, prevention is a major challenge, and today it has become one of the buzzwords of the entire health care system, which is struggling to deal with severe financial pressures. In mental illness, prevention depends on knowing what the risk factors are, and being able to intervene in time to do some good. Unfortunately, this dimension of clinical psychiatry is still poorly developed.

On the other hand, some of the most basic prevention situations are often quite obvious. One case study cited in the chapter on depression involved a single woman with three or more children under 10 who did not have a confidant. The risks built into her situation might be prevented with quite simple steps which could be taken by the community to improve her support system. Dealing with these conditions does not require extensive biochemical research, but merely the application of fundamental psychiatric knowledge clearly verified decades ago. The challenge is to actually execute these "simple" solutions, despite their sometimes being costly, because the payoff to society in terms of cost savings in the future might be enormous.

Another example stems from the reality that many mental illnesses are precipitated by stressful life events that initially produce anxiety. It is a reasonable step for the community to teach people stress management skills, perhaps as a normal part of a school curriculum. But whether such skills will actually lower the frequency of mental illness is not yet known.

There are also courses to help people learn how to be more assertive in coping with life problems — effectively assertive, not offensively aggressive. Individuals and families can also be taught about the life cycle and developmental changes we all undergo, so they can foresee transitions in their lives, then anticipate and plan for them.

While scientists have the capability to find solutions to major psychiatric illnesses in the coming decades, for better or worse, government policies and programs will be the most powerful determinants of the future of mental health and psychiatry.

In addition, adequate research funding is of course required. For example, we have seen that many of the more severe psychiatric problems may turn out to have relatively straightforward biochemical causes. Finding the underlying biological key to these problems would be enormously profitable to society, in terms of hard dollars, such as the costs of psychiatric institutions, legal processing, and the expensive involvement of numerous mental health professionals. But the soft dollar benefits might be far greater, when considering the lost productivity, creativity, and the reduced quality of family life of all those affected with schizophrenia, autism, depression, and so on.

Beyond scientific funding opportunities, it will also be helpful if the public can develop a broader understanding of the nature of mental illness. The public must have accurate information at hand in order to insist that various services, programs and treatments which have been clearly shown to be effective are given sufficient financial support to make them available to people who need them.

The references at the end of each chapter in this book can provide further information on each of the topics discussed. In addition, anyone having to deal with a severe mental illness, either personally, or in connection with a relative or friend, is encouraged to contact either the American or Canadian Psychiatric Associations for referrals to the most helpful and immediate sources of assistance:

- American Psychiatric Association: (202) 682-6000
- Canadian Psychiatric Association: (613) 234-2815

Index

D

E

F

G

H

I

L

M

N

O

P

Q

R

S

T

U

V

W

Contributors

Dr. Donald Addington (Depression)
Department of Psychiatry, Foothills Hospital, Calgary

Dr. Rudy C. Bowen (Anxiety and review of all chapters)
Department of Psychiatry, University Hospital, Saskatoon

Dr. John Bradford (Sexual Dysfunction)
Department of Psychiatry, Royal Ottawa Hospital, Ottawa

Dr. Evan Collins (AIDS)
Queen St., Mental Health Center, Toronto

Dr. John M. Cleghorn (Introduction & all chapters)
Departments of Psychiatry, McMaster University, Hamilton and University of Toronto

Dr. Charles Cunningham (Hyperactivity)
Department of Psychiatry, McMaster University, Hamilton

Dr. Benjamin Goldberg (Mental Retardation)
Department of Psychiatry, University of Western Ontario, London

Dr. Stanley Greben (Psychotherapy)
Department of Psychiatry, Mount Sinai Hospital, Toronto

Dr. Paul Grof (Depression)
Department of Psychiatry, Royal Ottawa Hospital, Ottawa

Dr. Nady A. el-Guebaly (Addictions)
Department of Psychiatry, University of Calgary, Calgary

Dr. Laurent Houde (Learning Disabilities)
Department of Child Psychiatry, Hopital du Haut-Richelieu, Saint-Jean

Dr. Steven Hucker (Sexual Dysfunction)
Forensic Service, Clarke Institute of Psychiatry, Toronto

Dr. Barrie Humphrey
Epidemiology and Psychiatric Services
Department of Psychiatry, McMaster University, Hamilton

Dr. Allan S. Kaplan (Eating Disorders)
Eating Disorder Clinic, Toronto General Hospital

Dr. Phillip Katz (Psychotherapy)
Department of Psychiatry, University of Manitoba, Winnipeg

Dr. David L. Keegan (Medical Disorders)
Department of Psychiatry, University Hospital, Saskatoon

Dr. Sidney H. Kennedy (Depression)
Department of Psychiatry, Toronto General Hospital, Toronto

Dr. Eddie Kingstone (Addictions)
Chairman, Department of Psychiatry, McMaster University, Hamilton

Dr. Nizar B. Ladha (Law)
Department of Psychiatry, Memorial University, St. John's

Dr. Saul Levine (overall critique)
Sunnybrooke Health Sciences Center, Toronto

Dr. Sebastian K. Littman (Deceased) (Schizophrenia)
Department of Psychiatry, University of Calgary, Calgary

Dr. W. John Livesley (Personality Disorders)
Department of Psychiatry, University of British Columbia, Vancouver

Dr. Brian J. McConville (Depression in Children)
Div. of Child and Adolescent Psychiatry, University of Cincinnati

Dr. Heather Munroe-Blum (Schizophrenia)
Dean, School of Social Work, University of Toronto, Toronto and
Department of Psychiatry, McMaster University, Hamilton

Dr. Hamish Nichol (Disorders in Children)
Department of Psychiatry, Vancouver General Hospital, Vancouver

Dr. D.R. Offord
Director, Child Epidemiology Unit
Department of Psychiatry, McMaster University

Dr. Gary Rodin (Depression in Medically Ill Patients)
Department of Psychiatry, Toronto General Hospital, Toronto

Dr. Isaac Sakinofsky (Suicide)
Psychiatrist-in-Chief, St. Michael's Hospital, Toronto

Dr. Mary V. Seeman (Schizophrenia)
Psychiatrist-in-Chief, Mount Sinai Hospital, Toronto

Dr. Brian F. Shaw (Cognitive Behavioral Therapy)
Psychologist-in Chief, Toronto General Hospital, Toronto

Dr. Kenneth Shulman (Alzheimer's Disease)
Department of Psychiatry, Sunnybrook Hospital, Toronto

Dr. Peter Szatmari (Autism)
Child Epidemiology Unit, Dept. of Psychiatry, McMaster University, Hamilton

Dr. Wendell W. Watters (Sexual Dysfunction)
Department of Psychiatry, McMaster University, Hamilton

Dr. Gabrielle Weiss (Hyperactivity)
Montreal Children's Hospital, Montreal

Dr. D. Blake Woodside (Eating Disorders)
Eating Disorder Clinic, Toronto General Hospital, Toronto

Dr. Donald Zarfas (Mental Retardation)
Children's Psychiatric Research Institute, London